# THE GOOD SLEEP GUIDE

Dr. Timothy J. Sharp is a qualified and registered clinical psychologist and a clinical academic in the University of Sydney's Department of Psychology, where he also coordinates the Good Sleep Program through the department's Clinical Psychology Unit. He is founder and director of Dr. Timothy J. Sharp & Associates and is involved in developing new programs and products for a range of clients.

For over a decade, Dr. Sharp has been helping people with psychological and medical problems in individual consultations and in group programs. His research, which has been published in scientific and academic journals locally and internationally, focuses on developing theories that better explain psychological problems and that lead to more effective methods of helping people. Dr. Sharp also gives talks to businesses and corporate groups about how to maximize work performance by ensuring the psychological health and well being of employees and by improving the work environment.

Dr. Sharp can be contacted at timothysharp@bigpond.com or you may wish to visit his web site at www.makingchanges.com.au.

# THE
# GOOD
# SLEEP
# GUIDE

*10 steps to better sleep*
*and how to break*
*the worry cycle*

## TIMOTHY J. SHARP
PhD, MPsych, BSc (Hons)

Frog, Ltd.
Berkeley, California

Published by Frog, Ltd.

Frog, Ltd. books are distributed by
North Atlantic Books
P.O. Box 12327
Berkeley, California 94712

First published by Penguin Books Australia Ltd. 2001

Book design by Debra Billson, Penguin Design Studio
Illustrated by Christina Miesen

Printed in Canada

North Atlantic Books' publications are available through most bookstores. For further information, call 800-337-2665 or visit our website at www.northatlanticbooks.com.

Substantial discounts on bulk quantities are available to corporations, professional associations, and other organizations. For details and discount information, contact our special sales department.

Library of Congress Cataloging-in-Publication Data

Sharp, Timothy James.
The good sleep guide: ten steps to better sleep and how to break the worry cycle / by Timothy J. Sharp.
        p. cm.
    Includes Index.
    Reprint. Previously printed by Penguin in Australia in 2001.
    ISBN 1-58394-075-8 (alk. paper)
    1. Sleep—Popular works.  I. Title.
RA786.S53 2003
616.8'498—dc21

2003004833

1   2   3   4   5   6   7   8   9   TRANSCONTINENTAL   08   07   06   05   04   03

*To my darlings,*
*Marnie and Tali*

# CONTENTS

# Acknowledgements

No publication is ever a solo effort and there are many to whom I am grateful for suggesting an idea or triggering a thought that eventually ended up in *The Good Sleep Guide*. I will mention only a few by name, but trust that the many others will know who they are and accept my sincere thanks.

First, were it not for my many patients and clients over the years this book would not have been written. I would also like to thank my academic and clinical colleagues (notably the staff and students who have helped to run the Good Sleep Program at the Clinical Psychology Unit at the University of Sydney) who have regularly challenged and inspired me to improve what I do and to work towards better ways of helping those in need. In particular, I would like to acknowledge the contribution of Dr. Michael Nicholas who has influenced my career in psychology more than anyone.

Specific mention also needs to be made of the team at Penguin Books Australia who from the first day I contacted them with the idea for this book have been marvelously supportive, encouraging and helpful. In particular, Julie Gibbs (Executive Publisher) and Heather Cam (Senior Editor) have shaped my ideas and my program into an accessible, easy-to-read guide.

Finally, I would like to thank my wife and my daughter, as well as all of my immediate and extended family, who daily provide me with the motivation to aim towards achieving bigger and better things.

# Introduction

Congratulations. You have taken the first important step in improving your sleep. One of the most common problems with sleep difficulties is that many people simply accept their lack of sleep, believing there is little or nothing they can do about it.

This sense of helplessness and resignation is unfortunate, because there are things you can do to get better sleep. *The Good Sleep Guide* outlines a program that has helped many people to sleep better and have a better life. The Good Sleep Program is based on proven coping strategies and innovative components and is effective.

## How *The Good Sleep Guide* will help you

One of the core assumptions of *The Good Sleep Guide* is that a healthy lifestyle contributes to healthy sleeping. It will consider a range of strategies to help you develop a healthier lifestyle which will, in turn, help you to sleep better. Topics covered include diet, exercise, relaxation and emotional well being.

 Remember: the key to healthy sleeping is a healthy lifestyle.

*The Good Sleep Guide* also addresses issues such as stress and time management, as there is little doubt that keeping your tension levels under control and organizing your days will assist with good sleep. You will learn different ways to relax, as relaxation helps you to get to sleep, as well as to generally manage better the stresses and challenges that you inevitably encounter during the day.

This guide outlines the most effective sleep strategies. These include developing a healthy sleep routine and avoiding some of the more common "bad habits" that can develop after not sleeping well for a while (such as napping during the day and trying to compensate for tiredness by drinking more coffee or using medications).

In addition, this guide tackles one of the most difficult of sleep-related problems, which is worry and racing thoughts. Worry is rarely addressed adequately in books on sleep or sleep programs, yet it commonly causes, and con-tributes further to, sleep-related problems. In most cases, overcoming worry requires more than relaxation skills. *The Good Sleep Guide* provides a proven and effective way of overcoming the "worry cycle," thereby significantly increas-ing your chances of getting good sleep.

 Chapter 8 shows you how to tackle worry and racing thoughts.

Finally, this guide includes information about related problems. Chapter 9 helps you determine if you are suffer-ing from one of the common psychological disorders that frequently accompany insomnia (such as depression or anx-iety) and reviews the most common treatments for these problems. At the back of the book in "Further help and some tips" are some guidelines for those wishing to seek fur-ther professional help. This section discusses several very specific sleep-related problems and issues (such as jet lag, shiftwork and new-born babies).

The Good Sleep Guide will help you:
- to understand sleep problems
- to assess your sleep needs
- to target potential problem areas
- to identify what you can do to improve your sleep.

## How to use this guide

I recommend that you work your way through the program one chapter at a time. If you think your problem essentially involves one specific issue, you may find it appropriate to go directly to a particular chapter. However, bear in mind that most of the sections are integrated and linked to other sections in the guide. A problem in one area will frequently create repercussions in another area. Therefore, the earlier chapters set the foundations for the later ones.

I am confident that if you work through the Good Sleep Program in a structured and committed way your sleeping will improve and you will enjoy life a lot more with your renewed vigour and new-found energy.

## Who will benefit?

Primarily, this guide is for those whose sleep problems cannot properly be accounted for by a specific medical problem. If you are not sure, then consult your doctor. Your doctor will also tell you whether or not it would be appropriate for you to visit a medical specialist and/or a specialist sleep clinic.

If you do have an identified medical problem, this guide may still be helpful. It often works extremely well in conjunction with other physical treatments, such as appropriate medications or CPAP (Continuous Positive Airway Pressure) machines. The reason is that these treatments, although helpful in some cases, do not always provide all the answers. There is nothing in this guide that can harm you. If you have tried everything recommended in this program and are still struggling to get the sleep you would like, then you might like to ask your doctor to reassess your condition and perhaps organize a specialist consultation. Your doctor or your sleep specialist may then be able to review what other options exist for you.

It is important to note that although the Good Sleep Program is an effective and successful one, it is not a miracle cure. It is based on the most up-to-date therapeutic practices and it is a proven intervention that has helped thousands of insomnia sufferers around the world. But, it is not necessarily a quick fix.

So, use this book as a guide, not a rule book. Every person is different and responses will vary. Individuals will therefore benefit from different aspects of the program. There are certain strategies that help some people, and may even change their lives. But these same strategies may have little effect on others. The only way to find out which ones will help you is to try them all. It's up to you to discover what works in your case.

Reading *The Good Sleep Guide* will not, on its own, improve your sleep. The success of this self-help program will depend on you doing more than just reading and thinking about the ideas and strategies presented. The success of this program will depend on you putting its recommendations into practice and then persevering for long enough to allow the program to work.

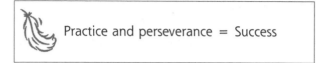

Practice and perseverance = Success

You can think of *The Good Sleep Guide* as being like a cookbook. You'll go hungry if you simply read it and think that the recipes sound nice or the pictures look good. You can, however, dine from the banquet of good sleep if you chose a recipe that suits you, gather the ingredients, and make the dish. Feel free to add salt and pepper to taste, but don't forget that the basic recipe is well established. There are many ways to bake bread, but you always need flour and water. The next ten chapters are the flour and water of an effective Good Sleep Program. The chapter titles give you the ten steps we will follow.

The ten steps to better sleep are:
1   Understand the need for sleep.
2   Make sleep a priority.
3   Watch your diet.
4   Exercise and be active.
5   Learn to relax.
6   Sort out your sleep routine.
7   Organize your time.
8   Develop healthy thinking and control worry.
9   Deal with other problems.
10  Persevere and practice.

# Meet Paul and Sonia

Before you begin the Good Sleep Program, there is one final formality. As you read the guide, you will encounter Paul and Sonia. I would like to introduce you to Paul and Sonia except I can't, because they don't really exist. Well, they do exist, but they are a composite of various people with sleep-related problems that I have seen and talked to over the years.

Paul and Sonia are also not perfect matches for you. Although this sounds obvious, it is important to remember, because there is a good chance that some of Paul's and Sonia's worries may not be exactly the same as the problems you are facing. Don't let this put you off. Just substitute your worries for Paul's and Sonia's. At the end of the day, a worry is just a worry and this book does not intend to deal with every specific one that you have, but rather to help you learn how to deal with them in general.

I have used Paul and Sonia in this way because it is simpler than using tens or even hundreds of names throughout this book. I believe it is important to provide real-life examples of problems other people have faced, but obviously I need to protect others' confidentiality.

So don't worry if Paul and Sonia appear to change in the course of this guide. Paul in Chapter 2 is not necessarily the same Paul as in Chapter 8. But, comprised as they are of bits and pieces of lots of people, I would be surprised if you did not discover aspects of yourself in Paul and Sonia—and do not forget that they have very real sleep problems, just like you do.

Most importantly you should remind yourself that this Good Sleep Program helped most of the Pauls and Sonias to sleep better. If you work your way through the next ten chapters and if you can implement the strategies outlined, then you too will start to experience the benefits that they have experienced. You too will start to sleep better and begin to realize how wonderful it is to sleep well and enjoy life.

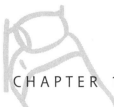

CHAPTER 1

# Understand the need for sleep

## Why is sleep so important?

Obviously you think sleep is important or you would not have started reading this book. There is a good chance you got this guide because you are tired, but sleep is not just important because it dispels tiredness. Sleep is important for many other reasons as well—being one of the cornerstones of health and well being. Unfortunately, this has not been widely acknowledged and consequently many people have suffered for too long with little guidance or help to overcome their problem.

> One of the foundation stones of health and well being is good sleep.

In the last few decades there has been an explosion of interest in diet and nutrition, as well as in activity and exercise. The benefits of healthy eating and regular activity are well recognized and widely accepted, not just by medical and health professionals, but also by the general community. This has been a fantastic advancement and a significant achievement for public health campaigners.

However, although many medical specialists and academics have tried to emphasize the importance of sleep, they have not had the same success in reaching the public. It is not widely known, for example, that good sleep is one of the most important components of healthy living. Not only has sleep missed out on the attention that nutrition and exercise have received, in some instances it has actually attracted negative publicity. Why does sleep have a bad reputation? People who eat well and ensure they have a balanced diet are respected for looking after their health. People who exercise regularly are admired for doing what we all know we should do (but often don't). But people who devote time to ensuring they achieve a good quality and quantity of sleep tend to be considered *lazy*!

In the 1980s and 1990s adequate sleep was discounted by many of the high-flyers as being unnecessary. A number of famous people were quoted as saying that they only needed a few hours of sleep each night. They often stated that sleep was a waste of time and that they would rather spend their time working and achieving success.

Well, that approach is fine if you can cope with only a few hours sleep each night. And some people can. A small percentage of people are able to get by with no ill effects on only three to four hours sleep each night. Some of these people are then able to use their extra waking time to work hard and achieve more. More's their luck!

But these people are definitely in the minority. For most people, three to four hours sleep each night is simply not sufficient and would cause sleep deprivation. (Seven to eight hours is the normal requirement.) Rather than freeing up more time to work, four hours sleep would produce tiredness and a range of symptoms that ultimately would affect the ability to concentrate and process information. Rather than allowing more time to achieve and succeed, it would cause most of us to struggle with the basics and barely be able to tie our shoelaces!

> A small percentage of people need no more than 3 to 4 hours sleep each night, but 7 to 8 hours is the normal requirement.

*The Good Sleep Guide*, therefore, is not about how to cope with minimal sleep or about how to achieve as much as possible while sleeping as little as possible. Rather, it is about helping you to get an appropriate and healthy amount of sleep, and a better quality sleep. In order to do this I believe it is important to make sleep more attractive—to make sleep "sexy!" Rather than shunning sleep, I argue that we should value it. Rather than trying to minimize sleep, we should recognize its restorative benefits and enjoy the beauty and tranquillity of restful slumber. As well as being a practical guide to help people to sleep better, *The Good Sleep Guide* aims to promote the significant benefits of sleep for individuals, relationships, work performance and productivity, as well as for society.

Sleep is not a vice. Cutting back or doing without may be a virtue if it's cigarettes, a second slice of mud cake, or nail-biting stress, but why cut back on something as healthful and restorative as restful slumber?

## The Good Sleep Guide can help you

I think I am probably safe in assuming that anyone reading this guide has experienced (or more likely is experiencing) disturbed sleep. Sleep problems are extremely common. For some people the problem is trouble getting to sleep, whereas for those who fall asleep without difficulty, their problem involves waking frequently through the night. For the lucky ones, a few bad nights is quickly followed by a return to their more typical pattern of restful slumber. For the not-so-lucky ones, those few bad nights can extend torturously into long and frustrating weeks, which in some cases then extend into depressing and disruptive years.

If this is your situation, do not despair. Achieving good sleep is possible. Even for those of you who might have had trouble sleeping for months or years, there is certainly hope. In fact, there is more than hope—there is an answer. Most sleep problems are very treatable. You do not need to go on suffering. You can achieve restful and peaceful sleep, just like many of your friends and family whom you currently envy. With good sleep comes improved mood and the energy and the ability to enjoy life more. Remember what it was like when you weren't so exhausted, tired and irritable? Well, you can be like that again—bright, happy and much more able to cope with life's stresses, as well as better able to enjoy life's bountiful opportunities. Just read on.

> Most sleep problems can be treated, so there is no need to go on suffering.

## Who else is not sleeping?

Sleep problems are as common as the common cold! Sleep problems affect almost everyone. Although not directly life-threatening, sleep problems can be extremely distressing and problematic. They are one of the hidden problems of our society and are also associated with an increased risk of illness.

Epidemiological research (the study of health and illness in large populations and communities) indicates that up to 80% of people have trouble sleeping at some stage in their lives. A large survey in the USA recently found that 58% of respondents reported some symptoms of insomnia. There is also good evidence to suggest that at least 20% to 30% of the population at large have significant, chronic (that is, longstanding) sleep problems. Think about those numbers: 80% of people, or eight out of every ten, have trouble sleeping at some stage in their lives.

You are not alone!
- 30% of people have serious sleep problems.
- 80% of people have trouble sleeping at some stage in their lives.

What these figures mean is that almost one-third of the people in your office are more tired than they need to be because of some serious sleep-related problem. One-third of the people in your street and in your neighborhood are tired and not getting enough sleep. One-third of the people on your bus or train are not sleeping well (you probably know the ones—those people whose heads nod forward and then jerk upward suddenly as they realize they are dozing off and are about to fall from their seats). More astounding is the fact that 80% of the population are experiencing short-term, minor problems.

## A brief overview of sleep disorders

But quoting these sorts of statistics only paints part of the picture. Although almost one-third of people sleep poorly, their sleep problems are not all the same. The terms "sleep disorders" and "sleep problems" cover a huge range of what, in some cases, might be very different problems. In one person, a sleep disorder might reflect a serious underlying medical condition. In another, a sleep disorder might be the result of a relatively benign (that is, relatively harmless) environmental stressor. Disturbed sleep and the frequently associated problem of tiredness might be indicative of sickness or of worry. There are many types of sleep problems and even more causes.

Health professionals (such as doctors and psychologists) who work in the field of sleep research and sleep therapy use a wide variety of terms to describe and label the many types of sleep problems. Among the terms, two specific ones are used more often than any others. Unfortunately, the two terms are often confused: "sleep disorder" and "insomnia" are not interchangeable terms. "Sleep disorder" is a broad term that covers all sleep-related problems. "Insomnia" refers to having difficulty falling or staying asleep, and to experiencing a poor quality of sleep. A quick overview of the most common sleep disorders will be helpful.

Historically, the medical and health systems in most Western societies have been based on ways of thinking that label problems and then divide them into categories. Doctors typically like to fit patients and their problems into "boxes." This also usually involves using very specific language and terminology to differentiate one "box" from another "box." Although not perfect, these systems and labels do help professionals to communicate with one another. If a sleep specialist refers to "obstructive sleep apnea," for example, another specialist will know exactly what they are talking about.

Several systems have been devised for defining and diagnosing sleep-related problems, but there are three major systems that have become particularly popular and that are now used in medical circles around the world. These three systems are known as:

1  the Sleep Disorders Codes in the Diagnostic and Statistical Manual of Mental Disorders (DSM)

2  the Sleep Disorders Codes in the International Classification of Diseases (ICD)

3  the International Classification of Sleep Disorders developed by the American Sleep Disorders Association.

Despite the fact that more than one system exists to label and diagnose sleep problems, there are several categories of sleep problems that are common to each of these three systems. For all intents and purposes there are three main categories of problems.

The first, *dyssomnia*, refers to problems falling asleep or staying asleep. The more commonly used term "insomnia" falls in this category, which also includes problems associated with poor sleep quality. Poor sleep quality refers to the phenomenon that although you have slept, you do not feel refreshed when you awaken.

The second category, *parasomnia*, refers to abnormal physiological or behavioral activities that occur during sleep. For example, some of the more common parasomnias include sleep walking (somnambulism), teeth grinding (or bruxism), and nightmares.

The third category of sleep-related problems includes those that are best explained by *medical disorders*. Conditions such as Parkinson's disorder, chronic obstructive pulmonary disease (COPD), asthma, and even some chronic pain problems (including arthritis and fibromyalgia) can all have sleep disturbance as a primary or secondary symptom. This group also includes sleep problems attributable to psychological disorders, such as major depressive disorder and some of the anxiety disorders, that also frequently have insomnia as a symptom.

If you would like to know more about these categorical systems you can find them and the codes (e.g. DSM and ICD) in your local library or on the Internet. These systems can be quite confusing since each of the codes uses slightly different diagnostic names and titles, as well as different groupings and subgroupings. Each code places more or less emphasis on different aspects of sleep disorders.

But even if you do understand the codes and even if you are able to "diagnose" your sleep problem, finding the right label for your sleep problem will not necessarily help you to fix it. For most of you, having a diagnosis should not necessarily affect the way you use this program. As will be emphasized more as you work through the book, for most, the best thing you can do is to slowly and gradually look at each recommended strategy and find out which ones work best for you.

## Insomnia

So we see that a diagnostic label is not always all that helpful since it does not always provide any guidance or any clues as to how to manage the problem. Knowing, for example, that you have insomnia and that your doctor refers to your insomnia as "idiopathic" or "psychophysiological" is unlikely to be all that helpful to you as you already know you are having trouble falling asleep. Having a name for our problems does not usually make them go away.

There are multiple and complex causes of insomnia. People from all walks of life come to me complaining of the same or very similar problems. For many people, such as Paul, the primary problem is getting to sleep or difficulty staying asleep.

*Paul came to me complaining that although he fell asleep without any problem (on most nights) he frequently woke at about 3 a.m. and often had difficulty getting back to sleep.*

*He reported that he would wake suddenly, only to find to his great irritation that his mind had clicked into gear and that he was already thinking about the day ahead. Although it was still early in the morning, Paul reported that he was not tired, and that his mind was actively mulling over the tasks and projects he would have to work on that day. Despite feeling relatively alert, he felt extremely frustrated. Paul reported feeling utterly perplexed that he was waking so early in the morning, when what he really wanted was to sleep another few hours before he needed to rise for work.*

*Sonia also reported problems staying asleep. Like Paul, she came to see me reporting that only very rarely did she have trouble falling asleep. Instead, she complained that she woke at least three or four times through the night. She reported that she would lie awake for up to thirty minutes before she could get back to sleep. Sometimes it would take her considerably longer. As a result, she stated that she felt tired when she got up in the mornings, as though she "never really obtained proper deep sleep."*

After careful assessment, it became apparent that although Paul's and Sonia's problems appeared somewhat similar (in that they both reported problems waking throughout the night), the causes of their problems were really quite different. Paul, I soon discovered, was waking early in the morning because he was going to bed too early and because he had unrealistic expectations about how long he could and should sleep.

*Paul would usually go to bed and turn off the lights at about 9 p.m. and expect to sleep until 6 a.m. This meant he was expecting to get about nine hours sleep, which is significantly more than most people really need (seven and a half hours is average). Thus, it was not surprising that he was waking at 3 a.m. as he had, by this stage, already had approximately six hours sleep. It turned out that this was only slightly less than his body needed.*

Most people spend, on average, 7½ hours asleep.

*Sonia, on the other hand, woke frequently throughout the night because her mind was constantly racing and she found it hard to stop continually thinking about her work. She admitted she had always been an anxious person and acknowledged that she had often found work stressful. She described herself as "a bit of a worrier." She had, however, been able to manage her stress until a recent promotion at work. Although she was proud of being offered this opportunity, she also found that it strained her resources and challenged her confidence. In order to avoid disappointing herself and her colleagues (not to mention her employers), she compensated by working extra hard and long. Unfortunately, this also contributed to extra worry that, in turn, affected her sleep.*

These cases provide just two examples of the many different causes of insomnia. One of the other more common problems is trouble falling asleep (as opposed to trouble staying asleep) which will be addressed in detail in Chapter 6. *The Good Sleep Guide* will examine *how and why* sleep problems come about and *what is maintaining them,* focusing on *what you can do about them.*

## Problems associated with insomnia

All too often sleep problems appear to be treated in isolation, with little or inadequate attention given to the consequences of chronic poor sleep and to the factors that may be maintaining poor sleep. Treating sleep problems without addressing these associated factors is like repeatedly recharging a car battery that keeps going flat without iden tifying why it is constantly losing energy. If, for example, you continue to leave your headlights on at night, the power will continue to drain away. Recharging the battery will only work temporarily, until you identify and modify this other contributing factor.

Any treatment that ignores these other factors, or any treatment that does not adequately address the whole range of physical, psychological and environmental problems that can contribute to insomnia, is a treatment that only addresses part of the problem. A partial treatment is bound to provide only a partial solution, and a partial solution is bound to fail or, at the very least, to leave you feeling unsatisfied. Failure is the last thing you want, especially if you have tried several treatments already and been disappointed.

Consider Paul, for example. His sleep problem had troubled him for more than six years by the time he sought treatment. This is not that unusual since a lot of people try to cope on their own and postpone their visit to a doctor or psychologist until they are at their wit's end. There are several reasons for this, but one of the more common reasons is that many people tend to think that insomnia is not a "real" problem or that it is not that "serious." It won't kill them and they have put up with it so far, so why go to the doctor? Alternatively, many people with chronic insomnia are simply too exhausted to seek help, or, in some cases, they are too busy trying to keep up with the daily demands made of them!

*Anyway, by the time Paul presented for treatment, as well as complaining of insomnia, he informed me that he had begun to feel more and more "down." He stated that he always felt tired during the day and consequently found it hard to enjoy things as much as he used to. He was more irritable than he used to be and tended to take out his bad moods on his wife— after which he felt very guilty. He also became more and more frustrated as he began to realize that his work performance was suffering. He found that he was making more mistakes at work and struggling to keep up with demand, whereas he had never had a problem with performance or productivity at work before. Because he was tired, he found it increasingly difficult to concentrate during important business meetings and while working on complex projects.*

*By the time Paul came to see me, therefore, he was not only suffering from insomnia. There is no doubt that he was not sleeping well, but he was also suffering from depression, irritability and frustration. He was experiencing problems at work due to tiredness, poor concentration and attention. As well as his work performance suffering, his marriage was beginning to be affected by his frequent angry outbursts. Although all of these problems might have started with his poor sleep, after many years of not sleeping well he had not just one problem but a number. Each was significant in its own right and contributed to other problems. It was essential, therefore, to address all of these factors to ensure success.*

Problems associated with insomnia have long been recognized and it is not a recent finding that depression can stem from insomnia. Some of these problems, however, do appear to be becoming more serious. In the 1990s a new disorder was identified and named in Japan. *Karo-jisatsu*, suicide from overwork, is increasing at an alarming rate among young to middle-aged Japanese males. More correctly, many of these men are killing themselves because of a lack of sleep. The long work hours are really only an indirect cause. In a celebrated and somewhat infamous case, a twenty-four-year-old man hanged himself after working for sixteen months with a large advertising firm in Tokyo. He had apparently become depressed after working outrageous and excessive hours. When his family successfully sued his employers, it was revealed that he had been sleeping for only thirty minutes to two hours each night and that he had not taken one day off in over a year.

 Karo-jisatsu means "suicide from overwork" (or, more accurately, suicide due to too much work and too little sleep and relaxation).

As highlighted in this particularly dramatic example, lack of sleep can inflict a terrible toll which at the extreme end of the spectrum can culminate in severe depression, even suicide. More commonly, the toll includes personal problems such as depression and irritability, difficulties at work, relationship troubles, tiredness, lethargy and even poor health. But a lack of sleep can also contribute to potentially disastrous problems that can affect the community at large.

A number of recent studies, mostly from the USA, have suggested that tiredness (usually stemming from sleep problems) may cause as many deaths on the road as does driving under the influence of alcohol. That this finding surprises so many people highlights the relative lack of attention given to a major life-threatening problem: tiredness induced by lack of sleep.

 Don't drive under the influence of alcohol, drugs, or tiredness.

Lack of sleep has also been blamed for several major catastrophes that have caused immeasurable damage to the environment and to society, as well as costing millions of dollars to remedy. Two of the more publicized disasters that were attributed to human error caused by tiredness are the *Exxon Valdez* oil spill and the *Challenger* space shuttle explosion.

Of even more relevance to most of you reading this book is the fact that every day, thousands, if not millions, of people around the world suffer injuries as a result of sleepiness. These injuries include those that are often experienced at work or in the kitchen, as well as on the road. These injuries, although not all ending in death, can still cause terrible suffering for the individuals involved and for their families. These injuries also cause considerable social and financial costs to the community (in the form of workers' compensation payments and increased insurance costs).

## Treatments for insomnia

There are literally hundreds if not thousands of treatments and remedies available—some dating back thousands of years, others developed more recently.

If you visit your local chemist, health food shop or even your local supermarket you will probably see a range of herbal remedies and over-the-counter medicines, as well as prescription drugs, all purporting to treat insomnia. Similarly, there are a bewildering number of books, cassette-tapes and videos that claim they will help you to overcome your problems. Some of these are valid interventions based on science and research. Others, however, are dubious as snake oil.

The aim of this guide is not to review and discuss all of the treatments on offer. Nor will I be recommending some treatments over others. I hope to help you work out which treatments (if any) are worth trying and which are best avoided. My main message is don't rush in and try everything and anything that proposes to deal with your problem. Don't believe every claim made on the packaging or in the marketing leaflets of various treatments. A healthy degree of skepticism is helpful. It is particularly important to carefully consider the possible side effects of medications and herbal remedies. Natural and herbal remedies are not necessarily safe just because they come from a plant or because they are not artificially produced by man.

Exercise a healthy degree of skepticism when it comes to herbal remedies. Not everything that is natural is automatically good for you: arsenic and opium, for example, are natural products, but both can be extremely dangerous and can kill.

I would encourage you to question your doctor, chemist, naturopath, psychologist or any other person treating you about the evidence for their particular treatment. Also it is important to find an appropriately qualified professional, especially if your insomnia is severe. Not every treatment is effective and not just anyone can help you overcome your sleep problem. There are good reasons why doctors and psychologists, for example, undergo formal registration in order to practice. It can be unsafe to provide some treatments without a sound knowledge of relevant medical and psychological theories and practices.

The simple truth is that many treatments on offer do not work. This is all the more frustrating when one realizes that there are effective and powerful treatments available. These treatments have been developed over many years by groups of clinicians, researchers and academics. They are effective and should be available to everyone who needs them. Insomnia is a very treatable problem and around eighty per cent of people suffering from insomnia can be helped. Nothing works all the time, but a good treatment should work most of the time.

> The strategies that make up the Good Sleep Program have been proven to work in trials conducted in treatment centers worldwide.

Many people I have seen professionally have tried numerous medications and expensive "miracle cures" before coming to me. Yet even after so many treatments and so many failures, they are still searching.

The good news is that there are strategies and treatments that work and that can help. *The Good Sleep Guide* is based on a tried and tested program. It is based on a well-established form of psychological therapy (known as "Cognitive Behavior Therapy" or CBT) that has withstood the test of time and the rigors of scientific analysis. Cognitive behavior therapy has been recognized by most of the relevant professional bodies around the world as being the treatment of choice for insomnia (as well as for a number of other related problems, such as stress and worry). The program outlined in this guide really works and has been proven to do so in numerous scientific trials in treatment centers all around the world. So happy reading and good sleeping!

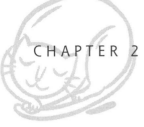

# CHAPTER 2

# Make sleep a priority

## The missing piece in the puzzle

Earlier I talked about making sleep "sexy," that is, improving its image and giving its many significant benefits more recognition.

 Make sleep a priority and watch your sleep improve.

For many years now, we have been educated about the benefits of a balanced diet and exercise. Quite rightly too.

For far too long, many people unwittingly contributed to their own poor health by eating products high in fats and salts, by eating too few fruits and vegetables, and by avoiding exercise.

The last decade or two has seen dietary information become available to the average person without a degree in nutrition or medicine, so that they can change eating habits for the better. Likewise, there has been a rapid increase in the recognition that regular exercise is beneficial for health and, as a result, more people are living better, healthier lives. It is these changes in our diet and activity levels, along with improvements in health care and medicine, that have contributed to increased longevity.

But there is something else that we spend more time doing than either eating or exercising—something that takes up almost one-third of our lives, yet receives virtually no attention: *sleep*! Sleep is the missing piece in the complicated puzzle that is health. The average person sleeps for seven to eight hours each night. That is far more time than anyone spends exercising (apart from an elite athlete). It is also substantially more time than anyone spends eating. It is also about as much time as many people spend working. In summary, it is more time than most of us spend on any other activity and yet it rarely gains a mention, it rarely rates a story and virtually never comes into consideration when people review what they could do to improve their life.

What takes up almost one-third of our lives, yet receives minimal attention? Sleep!

When people ask, "How can I be healthier?" the answer more often than not is "Eat better" or "Exercise more." Have you ever heard anyone say that to be healthier and happier you should sleep more or sleep better? Maybe when you were little and got cranky or sick your parents said, "Off to bed, you need more sleep. You are run-down and tired. Get some sleep and you'll feel better in the morning." But besides parents, sleep researchers and sleep clinicians, very few people recognize that sleep is a crucial piece of the health puzzle. Sleep is what helps us recuperate physically and psychologically. Sleep is when our energies are restored and when our memories and thoughts are organized and filed away. Sleep is the secret to, and foundation of, good health.

"Sleep . . . knits up the raveled sleeve of care,
. . . sore labor's bath,
Balm of hurt minds . . .
Chief nourisher in life's feast."
—William Shakespeare, Macbeth, II, ii

## ISN'T SLEEP A WASTE OF TIME?

If sleep were not important, then presumably we would have evolved into beings that did not require it. Think about how advantageous this would be. If we hadn't needed to sleep, we would have been less vulnerable to predators. We would now have more hours to enjoy ourselves, to spend time with friends and family, to travel, to learn a language or a new skill, to produce more, and to work and play harder.

So, isn't sleep a waste of time? No, we still sleep because sleep is essential and we all know it because we feel so good when we have been sleeping well. Even those of you who have been having difficulty sleeping for some time now will remember a time when you had a good night's sleep. If you can, you will also remember how good you felt when you woke. You might also remember how much more energy you had and how much more pleasure you gained from life.

# What happens when you don't sleep well?

When you don't sleep well there can be unpleasant and, at times, serious consequences. As noted earlier, poor sleep and tiredness have been blamed for several well-known disasters as well as countless fatal motor vehicle accidents.

People who are tired tend not to perform as well at tasks that require concentration and attention. Driving a car, operating machinery, performing surgery or any intricate job requiring dexterity and quick responses all demand concentration, coordination, and the ability to react quickly to unpredictable events. Making quick decisions can be extremely difficult if you are tired and finding it hard to concentrate. It is at these times that tired people are more likely to make mistakes. Unfortunately, in extreme cases, these mistakes can be fatal for themselves and others.

## STRESS AT WORK CAN LEAD TO STRESS AT HOME

Not all sleep-related problems have such potential for disaster. More generally, poor concentration and attention due to lack of sleep can affect work performance. This can lead to problems at work, such as criticism from employers and/or colleagues. Criticism is stressful. No one likes to be criticized, especially when you know that you are making silly mistakes due to tiredness. If only you could get some sleep!

Even if you are managing to hold things together at work, lack of sleep and chronic tiredness are frustrating, even depressing. Sometimes you feel like you can barely get through the day. Everything takes more effort. Nothing gives the same sense of pleasure or satisfaction. Over time, tiredness and exhaustion, combined with stress at work and lack of enjoyment outside of work, can contribute to excessive levels of suffering and even a sense of hopelessness.

Not surprisingly, these types of emotional problems have an effect on relationships. Many people become irritable when they are tired, and grumpy people are not good company. Partners who start off being understanding and supportive can, over time, reach the end of their patience.

Once a relationship begins to suffer, the stress and frustration only worsen. After a while, what started as a sleep problem can become a complex array of problems including lack of sleep, tiredness, difficulty concentrating and paying attention, depression, frustration, relationship problems and work performance problems. Without wanting to sound too negative . . . what a mess!

## Why not put more time into sleeping well?

Almost everyone agrees that good sleep is good. In fact, good sleep is wonderful, terrific, bliss. Good sleep can make almost any problem and almost any situation seem manageable. Good quality sleep can provide you with the strength and resources to cope with most of life's difficulties.

We also know that bad sleep is bad. In fact, bad sleep is terrible, it's torture. Bad sleep makes small problems appear insurmountable. Bad sleep turns molehills into mountains. Bad sleep robs you of energy and of enjoyment. Bad sleep takes away the ability to participate effectively and satisfactorily in life. Bad sleep affects your mood, your work, your relationships, your everything.

### "TREATMENTS" AND "CURES"

So why don't people do something about it? Well, usually they have. "I've tried," I hear you say, "but it hasn't worked." Both Paul and Sonia told me when I first saw them that they had tried a myriad of treatments and supposed "cures" in an attempt to get better sleep. Some of them had helped for a while, but none had really led to enduring or prolonged periods of good sleep.

When I first see someone I always assess the treatments that they have tried in the past. For many people this can be a long and extensive list, often including trials of tablets and herbs. It might extend to listening to some relaxation tapes or even undergoing acupuncture. Some people might have read a self-help book and/or seen a psychologist. But despite seeing several "experts" and trying several "proven treatments," the fact that they eventually came to see me suggests that they did not make as much progress as they would have liked. I assume that despite the treatments you have tried in the past, you too are not sleeping as well as you would like.

There are, however, those who have not tried anything before and, if this describes your situation, then great. I am confident that if you follow the program outlined you will be sleeping better within weeks.

But if you have tried lots of treatments before and they haven't worked as well as you would have liked them to, what do you do then? The first question I ask people in this situation is "Have you really done something?" By this I mean have you really made a significant effort to change your life? Have you really devoted yourself to making important changes, or have you just read a book, talked to a counselor, taken a few pills or herbal remedies? If sleep occupies a third of your life, and if you are not sleeping well, then let's say you may need to change about one-third of your life.

> Don't kid yourself that it's enough to just read a book, or talk to a counselor, or take a few pills or a herbal remedy. What *real* changes are you going to make to your lifestyle?

Now don't get scared. You don't need to change *everything*. *The Good Sleep Guide* is not about reorganizing every aspect of your life. And I would also like to add, I am not suggesting that you have not tried hard in the past. I am sure you have. But unfortunately many of the treatments you might have tried are simply not effective, so it is not your fault.

Now that you have found an effective program to implement, it is crucial that you are prepared to make some important changes to the way you do things and to the way you think about things

## MAKING A PERSONAL EFFORT IS THE KEY

For the Good Sleep Program to work, *you* need to make it work. Some people are not prepared to do the hard yards, to put in the time and the effort, to make this program work. Curiously, most people realize that to get fit, they need to exercise regularly. They know that no one else, not even a personal trainer, can get fit for them. Similarly, to lose weight most people realize that they need to watch how much they eat and what they eat. Other people (say a dietitian) can advise them of what a balanced diet includes, but they can't eat (or not eat) foods on another's behalf. But despite taking responsibility for their own exercise program or diet, many people expect that someone else or something else (such as a tablet) will fix their sleep problem. These people are usually disappointed when this approach is not effective.

So you must not expect me to do the work of "curing" or "fixing" your sleep problem. As much as I would like to, it simply is not possible. For most chronic insomnia sufferers there is only one person who can "fix" their sleep. I can guide you through this book and if you are still struggling you could go to see an expert (such as a clinical psychologist or a sleep doctor), but even then success will almost certainly depend on you following their advice.

"OK," I hear you say, "tell me what to do and I'll do it. I'll do anything to get better. Just show me the way." Well, that is a good start.

*Paul said those very words when he first came to see me, but after a few weeks he still was not sleeping well. He had experienced a few nights when his sleep was better, especially when he tried a few of the strategies that he had not tried before, but overall there was no significant improvement. After a careful analysis, it became apparent that he was not consistently applying the strategies. When we discussed this he told me that, although they seemed to help him, he did not have time to do them every day.*

*He did not have time! Paul had been experiencing insomnia for over twenty years. He was frustrated and irritable. He was still performing relatively well at work, but his domestic and social life were not nearly as good as they could have been. His evenings and weekends were mostly occupied with trying to catch up on lost sleep. He was sick and tired (literally) of not sleeping well, but couldn't find the time to make it better! Unfortunately, Paul's sleep did not improve very much at this stage because, despite his distress and despite the negative consequences he repeatedly complained of, for various reasons sleep was not as important to him as his work. As much as he said he wanted to sleep more and to sleep better, doing something about his sleep always came second to his work demands.*

This is one of the most common reasons why more people don't do more to sleep better. Because at the end of the day other things are more important. For all its problems, lack of sleep on its own won't kill you. So even if your sleep problems continue, you'll survive.

## BUT IS SURVIVAL ENOUGH?

Do you want to live the rest of your life in a haze of exhaustion? Don't you think that there must be a way of enjoying life more? Of participating more? Of being alive more? Just try to imagine the joys and benefits of having more energy, more tolerance and of being able to think more clearly on a regular basis.

"Of course I want this," I hear you say again. And I know that you probably would not be reading this book if you did not want to sleep better and if you did not realize that there might be benefits to sleeping better. But how important is sleep to you *really*? How much do you value sleep? What are you prepared to do about it and are you prepared to consider making changes to your daily routine, your nightly routine, and to your home and work situations?

> What are you willing to commit to in order to prove how very much you really do value good sleep?

If you don't have the time to devote to sleeping, you won't sleep well. If you don't value sleep, you will never make the effort to achieve good sleep. If you view sleep as a negative activity, as a waste of time, you will probably never sleep well (or sleep enough). It is important to recognize the damage that some of these misconceptions can inflict. Needing more than four hours sleep is not a sign of laziness or weakness. It is more accurately a demand of your biological make-up.

Rather than being a sign of laziness, getting good sleep can actually help you to succeed and achieve more. You are unlikely to perform well if you are tired, irritable, and fuzzy-headed. Successful people don't usually complain that they are exhausted every day. Healthy and happy people are generally healthy and happy because they do sleep well. If you make sleep a priority and if you achieve good sleep, then you too can be healthy, happy and successful in what you do.

## Make sleep a priority

As we already know, getting good sleep can eliminate, or at least significantly reduce, most of the frustrating and unpleasant problems that accompany insomnia. Getting good sleep can, in fact, do a lot more. Getting good sleep can help you to feel better physically and mentally. Getting good sleep can help you to feel happier, make you easier and more fun to be with, let you regain your energy. Good sleep can enable you to perform better at work. Better performance can lead to increased job satisfaction and to promotions. Good sleep can be good all round.

But achieving good sleep requires making an effort and treating your sleep as a priority. Getting good sleep requires perceiving sleep as a desirable, necessary goal and not as a waste of time. If sleep has to take second place to other things, then it will continue to be problematic. Although it is understandable that many people put other things (such as work) first, this might actually be part of the reason why they are having sleep problems. Devoting some time and energy to overcoming insomnia will help, not interfere with, your work and other areas of your life that you value. When you are sleeping better you will almost certainly be able to concentrate and focus better, and you will feel better, make decisions more effectively, and generally cope and function at a higher level.

So concentrating on getting better sleep will allow you to focus more on other enjoyable and necessary tasks and duties. Making sleep a priority will enable you to succeed in other areas. Good sleep is the foundation upon which you can build your successes.

You will need to put in some hard work in order to reap the rewards of victory. You need to devote time to practicing and applying the strategies described in this guide. They are necessary for you to get good sleep.

> We know that in sport victories do not just happen—a win is actually the result of weeks, if not years, of practice and training. So too with sleep.

## Determine to do something

The key to success is doing something. What *you* do will be the most influential variable in this program.

I am referring essentially to your behavior, your lifestyle. As will be discussed more in the coming chapters, there are a range of lifestyle factors that affect the way you sleep. What you eat can affect your sleep, as can how much you eat, and when you eat. How active you are can influence your sleep. Being generally active throughout the day can be helpful. Intensive exercise on a regular basis can also make a difference, depending on what you do and when you do it. Regular relaxation and having fun are other "lifestyle" activities that can make a significant difference.

Doing the things that will help you to sleep better will also involve doing what will help you to feel better, happier and more relaxed, things that you might not be doing now.

What all of this means, therefore, is doing some new things. Or alternatively, not doing something you are doing now. *You will need to make some changes.* Change is not impossible. We can all change. We all do change. Mostly, we change the way we do things if and when something becomes important enough. And this comes back to making sleep a priority. If you really want to get good sleep and if you really want to experience the benefits of good sleep (such as feeling better and happier, not to mention having more energy and performing better at work), then you need to see sleep as a priority. Sleep should be considered as important as a good diet and regular exercise. Sleep should be considered to be as important as almost any other aspect of your life.

 Sleep is as important as a healthy diet and regular exercise.

People can achieve all sorts of difficult goals when

something means enough to them. I've seen long-term, chronic smokers who have failed at numerous attempts to quit, successfully give up when they decide to have a baby. Or people with drinking problems abstain following a near-fatal motor vehicle accident. I have also seen gamblers stop throwing money down the drain once their partner has threatened to leave them.

Unfortunately, not everyone succeeds in their endeavors to achieve these goals and, even those that do, do not always find it easy. Changing the way we do things can be hard, especially if what we are trying to change is a long-term habit. In some cases what you might be trying to change is years of learning (what psychologists refer to as "conditioning"). Clearly, this will not always be easy, but it can be made easier if you are determined to make your goal (that is, sleeping) a priority. Achieving change can be made easier if you are determined to work hard at it.

## Commit to the program

This is where some people fail. Caught up in the demands of the present, they lose sight of the long-term goal. Given that experts have estimated that only one in five people sleeps well *without any effort*, that means four in five either don't sleep well or have to work at sleeping well. It is a myth that sleep does or should come easily.

Yet many of those four in five people are able to find ways to improve their sleep and to sleep better. They sleep well because they make an effort. And if something is important enough, and if the gains are worth it, making that effort can be very rewarding. Think how good it would be to sleep well. It can happen. *You* can make it happen.

When I first begin to treat someone, I always spend the first few sessions addressing this issue. If you don't decide to make sleep a priority and if you don't decide to commit to the program, then reading the rest of this guide will be a waste of time. Making the changes suggested in *The Good Sleep Guide* might be difficult. But they will be less difficult if you have spent time on this early, but crucial stage of the program.

> When Paul first came to see me and I began to ask him how important gaining good sleep was and whether or not he was willing to commit to the Good Sleep Program, his initial reaction was to feel insulted. He found it hard to believe that I would question his commitment and dedication. He was upset that I did not believe that he would act on the program's recommendations. At one point in our discussion, Paul said to me "I'm here, aren't I?" suggesting that his presence in my rooms was an indication that he was motivated and ready. Later he attempted to explain why he was upset, referring to the fact that he thought I was suggesting he had not tried in the past. Paul said, "I'm so committed to this . . . I want to sleep so badly that I've tried almost every sleep treatment in this city."

Although I certainly did not intend to insult Paul, I did intend to assess his motivation and his willingness to commit to the program. I did so because I consider this first step to be the most important step. Coming to see a psychologist or a doctor or any health professional is not enough—not on its own. Turning up for your appointment for an hour a week is relatively easy. Going home and doing what is necessary outside of my rooms and making the lifestyle changes that are needed is the hard part.

People who have tried "every treatment" are not necessarily committed or motivated. More likely they are desperate. It may be an indication that the person wants to be fixed, but it is not necessarily a sign that they are willing to do something themselves to bring this about—beyond going to a doctor or psychologist, which is not enough. It is *what you do* at home that will make the difference. "But I did try what they suggested," Paul replied. "For almost a week I did exactly as I was told, and it made no difference." Unfortunately, this is an all-too-common reply from people who have tried lots of "treatments." When I hear this I realize how important it is to commit to the program for a reasonable period of time.

## WHAT'S A REASONABLE PERIOD OF TIME?

Well, it is hard to give a definite answer because it varies from person to person. But, on average, for most people who have had sleep problems for months or years, it can take four to six weeks to realize some significant benefit. If you are lucky you might begin to experience gains sooner, nevertheless it is important to commit to the program for at least four to six weeks so that the benefits and changes are given time to consolidate. After that period of time you can experiment and you might be able to ease off some of the more restrictive parts of the program. However, for most people, the benefits will only last as long as they continue to apply and finetune those strategies that have helped them.

If you are prepared to work hard and commit to the program outlined in *The Good Sleep Guide* you will experience all the wonderful benefits associated with sleeping well. To experience these benefits:

1 You need to commit to the program.
2 You need to do what is recommended.
3 You need to keep doing what has helped.

## Still unsure?

If you are still unsure whether you are willing to commit to the program for the next four to six weeks, you might want to consider the following issues. Following this, I would encourage you to try the exercise at the end of this chapter.

### IS IT THE RIGHT TIME FOR YOU TO COMMIT?

If you have too many things on at the moment, or if your life is disrupted or unsettled by something in the short term, it might be better to wait until you have a period of four to six weeks when things will be relatively stable.

*Sonia, for example, first came to see me three weeks before her wedding. After her wedding she was having a honeymoon for two weeks. Obviously, it would not have been sensible or appropriate to start the program then and there. She was ready, but we agreed that it would be more reasonable to begin when she returned from her holiday, as she would almost certainly be in a better position to focus on what she needed to do.*

So think about whether now is the right time for you and whether or not you can give the program adequate attention. However, if your life is always hectic and you are constantly in a state of flux, waiting for the "right time" might mean waiting forever. In this case, you might need to assess your life in more general terms before you address your sleep problem (if this applies, you'll probably find it worthwhile having a look at Chapter 7 on time management).

> Give yourself a fair chance. Wait until there's a stretch of 4 to 6 weeks in which you can properly implement the program.

## DO FOUR WEEKS SEEM LIKE A LONG TIME?

Ask yourself how long you think you could commit to the program. If you can commit yourself to two weeks, or even one week, that might be a start, but don't expect too much. It might be better than nothing, but you probably won't get the full benefit and so may be disappointed. Think about another problem and ask yourself how long it might take to master a skill or to achieve significant change in some other area of your life. Losing weight and keeping weight off, for example, frequently takes at least six to twelve months. Getting fit in the gym often takes at least three to six months. Learning to type can take several weeks, if not months, of intensive practice. Developing new skills and learning new strategies can take time, but it is usually worthwhile. Compared to acquiring these other skills or compared to making these other changes, setting aside four to six weeks to improve your sleep is not necessarily a long time. And there is potentially even more to gain!

## THINK OF WHAT YOU HAVE TO GAIN

In fact, don't just *consider* it, write it down. Pull out a pen and some paper:

1 List all the reasons you bought this book.
2 List all the reasons you want to sleep better.
3 List all the benefits you hope you'll gain once you start to sleep well.
4 List all the things you don't like about being tired and hate about not sleeping well.

Write in big, clear letters and stick the lists next to your bed. Read them often. Doing this can help to develop the sort of motivation needed to tackle this demanding, but highly successful, program. Establishing this sort of motivation is the first step to succeeding with *The Good Sleep Guide*.

# CHAPTER 3

# Watch your diet

## You are what you eat

As you already know, diet is an important contributor to your health and to your general well being. The old saying "you are what you eat" means that if you eat well and you consume a sensible, balanced diet of nutritious foods, you will be healthy. If, on the other hand, you eat unhealthy, fatty foods with a high salt content, you are more likely to be unhealthy and to suffer illnesses.

What you may not have realized is that diet and nutrition can also influence your sleep. So, what you eat is an important part of your lifestyle that might be worthwhile reviewing. Although there are many old wives' tales referring to certain foodstuffs that supposedly assist or, alternatively, impair sleep, there is little scientific evidence to support these claims. Such claims are often inconsistent and contradictory, with some endorsing consumption of products such as garlic, teas, and meats, while others recommend avoiding them at all costs!

So this section of *The Good Sleep Guide* is not about recommending or advising against *specific* foods. To do so would be conjecture and not based on reliable research or even on consistent clinical experience. Rather, as stated already, this guide is based on the assumption that healthy living will contribute to healthy sleeping. So what follows is not a magical sleep-inducing diet, but some basic suggestions regarding healthy eating.

> This chapter also covers the issues of medication use, alcohol and caffeine consumption, and smoking.

## A balanced diet

A balanced diet is something that everyone should aim for since the benefits in the short term and in the long term are considerable. A balanced diet can lead to an enhanced sense of well being, including increased levels of energy and better sleep. Achieving a balanced diet basically involves ensuring that you consume adequate amounts of each of the major food groups on a regular basis and consume a variety of foods. For example, although it is generally recommended that you avoid too many fats and sugars, these are still necessary and important, in moderation.

## MODERATION IS THE KEY

Most foods are not too bad for you if eaten in moderation. There are some foods, however, that you should try to eat more of, and others that are best kept to a minimum. Specifically, the majority of your diet should comprise breads, cereals, fruits and vegetables. The most important categories of food are the fruits and vegetables; these provide the most dietary advantages and, typically, people don't consume enough of these life-enhancing foods.

It is also important to ensure that you eat adequate protein. Protein is to be found in red meat (such as beef and lamb), as well as white meat (such as fish and chicken). This group also includes dairy products. Some people think that they should avoid foods such as milk, cheese and yogurt, because they believe they are high in calories and will make them fat. That is only partly true. Some of these products are relatively high in calories, but they also include important and necessary vitamins and calcium that we need if we are to be healthy.

Eat a balanced diet.

Finally, it is important to eat small amounts of fats, oils and sugars. Butter, margarine, oils (particularly polyunsaturated ones) and sugar are essential parts of a well-balanced diet. Their consumption should be restricted because they provide few nutrients, while being relatively high in kilojoules, but remember that the secret is balance. Because you don't need a lot of this group of foods, you rarely, if ever, need to add them to your diet. If, for example, you eat a good balance of the other food types mentioned, you will, within these foods, already be consuming enough fats and oils for your needs.

## HOW MUCH TO EAT, AND WHEN?

In addition to eating a variety of foods from each of the major food groups every day, it is also generally recommended that you have several small- to medium-sized meals in preference to one large meal. Try to spread your consumption across the day, perhaps adding morning and afternoon snacks (such as a piece of fruit or some vegetable sticks) to your three (small to moderate) meals. Leave the banquets and feasts for those rare special occasions!

Although I do not believe that there are any specific foods that enhance or impair sleep, there are a few specific suggestions relating to sleep that you should consider besides the general recommendations for a balanced diet. For example, most specialists recommend that you avoid eating too close to bedtime and that you avoid having too large a meal, particularly late at night. Generally, it is recommended that your main meal should be in the middle of the day and that your evening meal should be smaller and lighter.

At the same time, it should be acknowledged that this "ideal" advice is not practical for many people. Most people prefer to have their main meal in the evenings because it is the only time of the day when they can sit down with their family or friends to eat together. Also the evening meal probably is the one meal they can enjoy slowly, without worrying about rushing off to, or back to, work. Whatever the reason, if you prefer to have a substantial and leisurely evening meal, try to ensure it is not too late. As a rule of thumb, you should try to leave at least two hours between the end of your evening meal and settling down to sleep.

Some people complain that spicy or rich foods in the evening cause them indigestion or stomach problems which waken them in the night. If this is your experience, then it might be best to skip these types of food for a while to see if it helps. But if chilies and curries don't trouble you, by all means eat them—in moderation.

## Alcohol

"Diet" can include anything that you eat, drink, swallow and consume, so let's consider alcohol intake. The use of alcohol (the "nightcap") to try to get to sleep is extremely common. This is not surprising since in Western societies alcohol is a widely accepted form of self-medication—that is, many people use it not just for social occasions and for enjoyment, but to deal informally with stress, anxiety and even sleep problems.

Another reason why alcohol is used to induce sleep is that it can actually work. Consuming one or two drinks with or after dinner in the evenings can have a sedative effect. Yet many people who have an evening drink, or two, continue to experience sleep difficulties.

> When Paul first came to see me and underwent the usual assessment I conduct when I first meet a new client, he acknowledged that he drank at least one or two glasses of wine each night with dinner. Paul swore by the "fact" that these drinks helped him to unwind after a busy and stressful day and that they helped him to get to sleep. However, he complained bitterly that he was not sleeping well, that he had not slept well for over ten years and that he couldn't cope any longer unless he was helped to get more sleep.
>
> Paul provides a classic example of someone persisting with a strategy (in this case, drinking) despite their problem (insomnia) not getting any better. For all intents and purposes, the strategy was not having any long-term beneficial effect.

So how do we understand a person's belief that alcohol is helping them when they continue to experience trouble sleeping, as well as all the associated difficulties of being tired?

The answer lies in the paradoxical effects of alcohol. Alcohol is what is known as an anxiolytic or a sedative. This means that it can be relaxing (as no doubt we can all confirm!). This relaxing effect, however, only occurs at certain doses. Once you consume more than a relaxing dose, alcohol can become disinhibiting and can begin to be quite stimulating. Anyone who has ever drunk more than they should have has experienced this very common effect. Although the level at which the change occurs varies for different people, almost all of us who drink alcohol have experienced feeling relaxed after one to two drinks, then excited, aroused, more confident and apparently more alert after three, four or more drinks.

So one of the important factors to keep in mind here is not just whether or not you drink at night but *how much* you drink. Drinking small amounts may actually assist sleep. Drinking within the safe, recommended levels might be OK (that is, one to two standard drinks for women and three to four standard drinks for men). A standard drink, for example, is a middy of beer (not a schooner), a small glass of wine, or a nip of spirits (which in most cases is approximately one bottle cap). Also it is recommended you don't drink every day (or night), but confine your alcohol consumption to four or five days a week.

There are two other aspects of alcohol consumption that you, as a sleeper, need to consider. One is that if you are drinking moderate to large amounts of liquid (any liquid) late at night, you will probably need to empty your bladder some time in the early morning. Waking with a full bladder can be uncomfortable and, not surprisingly, can disturb your sleep. Further, alcohol is metabolized by our bodies within several hours of consumption. When alcohol is being broken down, withdrawal-type symptoms can occur. These can include physiological arousal (e.g. increased heart rate and sweating) which not surprisingly can interrupt sleep. So although one or two drinks a few nights each week might not be a problem, regular excessive drinking can affect sleep by requiring you to go to the toilet and/or by causing withdrawal-type symptoms that can be arousing.

Finally, and more generally, excessive drinking contributes to poor health and even to depression, neither of which is likely to be associated with good sleep. If you are drinking considerably more than the safe, recommended levels noted above, then you should probably consider seeking specialized, professional help. Similarly, if you are drinking regularly and feel that you couldn't possibly sleep without a drink, then you should consult your local doctor. If you are in this category, it is unlikely you will be able to conquer your sleep problem until you have overcome your drinking problem. It is possible to learn how to control a drinking problem, so I strongly encourage you to seek help now.

## Sleeping pills

If you are taking sleeping tablets, they may be a benzodiazepine (such as Valium and Normison), an antidepressant (such as Tryptanol, Prothiaden, Prozac or Zoloft), or an antihistamine (such as Phenergan). Or you may be using one of the over-the-counter medications for which a prescription is not needed.

Each of these medications works in a different way and has a distinct effect. Each has some advantages and some disadvantages. In the short term, for transient sleep problems that do not have a long history, taking medications for a limited amount of time can be helpful and relatively problem-free. However, if you have a longstanding sleep problem and you have been taking medications for a long time (e.g. for more than four to six weeks), then you should carefully assess how effective these drugs really are.

If you have been using a medication to try to sleep and if you are still experiencing problems with your sleep, then it is likely that the medication you are taking is not working. You might fear that your sleep would be even worse without the medication, but many people actually think their medications are doing far more than they really are. Similar to Paul and his nightly alcohol consumption, if you think your medications are working, then why isn't your sleep better and why are you reading this book?

> For example, when Sonia came to see me she had been taking a benzodiazepine medication (also often referred to as a 'sedative' or 'hypnotic') for many years. Despite this, she reported not sleeping well—for many years. She continued to take the tablets every night, however, because she believed they were helping her get to sleep and that without the tablets she would "never get any sleep at all". But curiously, she had

*never really tested this belief and for several years had never seriously tried to sleep without the medication.*

*Sonia reported that she had tried to stop taking the drugs on a few occasions, but only for one or two nights and then, when she did not sleep well, she resumed taking the tablets. Because it takes longer than one or two nights for your body to clear itself of the medication and adjust, this does not represent a fair or adequate trial. There is also the matter of the withdrawal you inevitably experience if you have been taking medications for a while and then stop. These can be very mild in most cases, but still sufficient to disrupt your sleep for more than a couple of nights. Therefore, it is not surprising that Sonia did not sleep well for the first few nights. Her body was undergoing changes and getting used to not having the drug. If she had persisted, however, this would have settled within a few more days and she would almost certainly have begun to get better sleep.*

---

Remember it takes at least a few nights for your body to rid itself of any sleeping medications you have been taking. Allow time for your body to adjust.

---

I'm not suggesting you should stop taking all of your medications at once, because for some people this could be dangerous. I am, however, suggesting that you think carefully about whether the medications are helping or not and, if they are not helping, you consider gradually reducing your use of them. If you do decide that you are interested in reducing your dependence on medications, then I strongly advise you to consult your local doctor or specialist first. They will tell you whether you can just stop straightaway, or whether you would be better to gradually reduce your intake, slowly, over a few weeks. They might also decide, depending on the drugs you are taking, that it would be helpful to monitor you during the reduction phase.

## SIDE EFFECTS OF MEDICATION

As well as the possibility that the medications may not actually be helping all that much, there are other reasons you should consider ceasing to use them in the long term. One reason is that all medications have side effects. Despite what some people think there is really no such thing as a perfectly "clean" medication. Some are more harmful than others, but all medications will, over time, have some impact on your inner organs and on your health. Many medications affect your liver and kidneys. Some of these effects are permanent, although most are temporary and your body will recover once you cease the medication. Some of these medications also have cognitive and emotional effects of which many people are not even aware. That is, many of them affect your thinking, your ability to make decisions, and your mood. Some of the sedative medications cause a hangover in the morning. Some of them lead to people feeling groggy. Others can cause significant levels of drowsiness during the day.

> All medications have side effects.

If you have been taking sleep medication for more than a few weeks (and especially if you have been taking it for more than a few months), then it is likely you are experiencing side effects as a result of your medication. You may not actually be aware of these side effects as they can be subtle (some only become apparent after several years, or when you stop taking the medication and notice feeling different). Whether you are aware of them or not, these side effects might be slowly, but significantly, affecting your general health.

## DRUG TOLERANCE AND DEPENDENCE

Some medications also lead to you developing tolerance and/or dependence. This occurs when your body gets so used to the drug that it relies (or becomes dependent) on it. At the same time, the drug becomes less effective (and the body more tolerant of the drug) and larger doses are needed to gain the same effect. Once dependence occurs, your body can become distressed if it doesn't have a sufficient supply of the drug in its system. This distress is known as "withdrawal," and in some cases is extremely unpleasant. A similar phenomenon affects smokers and heavy drinkers when they try to break their habit. People who have become dependent on sleep medications can develop a problem known as "rebound insomnia."

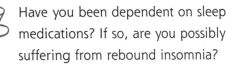

Have you been dependent on sleep medications? If so, are you possibly suffering from rebound insomnia?

Because many of the sleep-related medications lose their effectiveness when used regularly over a long period of time, people tend to increase their dose in order to achieve the same results. Eventually, there is no higher dose for the person to take and at this stage people either need to find a new medication or the medication simply becomes ineffective. After a while, this can contribute to worsening sleep. People in this situation become trapped in a vicious circle, in which their sleep problem actually worsens despite taking considerable and increased amounts of medication.

## MEDICATION FOR THE SHORT TERM ONLY

Despite what many people think, medications are frequently not the answer to long-term sleep problems. If you can take a medication for a few weeks and it helps to restore good sleep, that's fine. But that's the point at which you would be advised to stop. Medications can have a useful and important role to play if used appropriately and early, and if discontinued after a relatively short period of time. But if you are still having problems after using medications regularly for longer than three to four weeks, you should probably talk to your doctor about gradually reducing the medication and trying other strategies.

The program outlined in *The Good Sleep Guide* can be an effective replacement for medications and, in the long term, the strategies recommended in this guide will be far more effective (without the negative side effects). But remember, if you are thinking of ceasing or reducing your medications, consult your doctor first and get professional advice about how best to achieve your goal and cope with the possibility of short-term withdrawal effects.

 Consult your doctor before going off or reducing your medications.

## Caffeine

What you drink can affect your sleep as much as what you eat. Most notably, products that contain caffeine are stimulants and are likely to have an impact on the quality of your sleep, especially if consumed in large quantities and/or if consumed too close to sleep times.

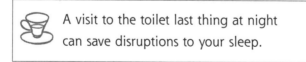 A visit to the toilet last thing at night can save disruptions to your sleep.

Drinking caffeine products can disrupt your sleep in at least two ways. One being that if you drink a lot late at night you are simply more likely to need to go to the toilet. If you are already having problems sleeping, you don't want to do anything that might disrupt your sleep. The simple solution is to avoid drinking too much liquid (especially caffeinated drinks and alcohol) late at night and make a practice of going to the toilet just before you go to bed.

Caffeine can also affect your sleep because it is a stimulant. Stimulants are drugs that cause mental and physiological arousal. Stimulants can contribute to increased activity inside your body and your mind, which will tend to keep you awake and interfere with your sleep.

The most commonly consumed caffeine product is coffee. It is hard to provide a safe level of consumption because the strength of caffeine in coffee varies considerably depending on whether you are drinking instant coffee or the usually much stronger espresso, brewed from freshly ground beans and produced by a commercial coffee machine. Taking this variation into account, it is probably unwise to drink more than two to four cups of coffee each day. Also, it is probably best not to drink coffee after about 5 p.m. or 6 p.m. Some people go further and argue that you should not drink any coffee after 3 p.m. or 4 p.m., since caffeine is active and in your system many hours after you have drunk it. Given this, an after-dinner coffee consumed around 6 p.m. or 7 p.m. may impair your ability to get to sleep at 10 p.m. or 11 p.m.

 Keep your coffee intake down to 2 to 4 cups daily. Avoid drinking coffee after 5 p.m.

Additionally, it is important to take into account that people are affected very differently by drugs, including caffeine. Some people can drink a cup of coffee and go to bed, falling asleep several minutes later. Others will experience a "buzz" and a sense of heightened arousal (including increased mental alertness) for several hours after drinking. If you are not sure to what extent coffee is affecting you, cut back on it or stop drinking it altogether, especially in the evenings, and see what happens. One caution, however: remember that caffeine is a drug and so, if you have been a long-term heavy user, cutting it out all at once can lead to headaches, agitation, irritability, tiredness, difficulty concentrating, and other similar withdrawal symptoms. If you have been drinking a lot of coffee and you want to reduce your consumption or cease altogether, it might be useful to consult your local doctor first.

Remember too that coffee is not the only product that contains caffeine. Caffeine is also present in tea (although there are many herbal, non-caffeinated teas available), chocolate (including chocolate drinks), many soft drinks (particularly colas and some of the new "energy drinks"), and even some medications. If unsure, check the ingredients or labels of the products you are consuming. You may be surprised to find that you are consuming stimulants without realizing it.

*I once saw a young man who complained of sleep problems and who revealed, after I had asked him a number of questions, that he was drinking over three liters of soft drink each day. Apart from the other effects this was almost certainly having on his health (considering, among other things, the high sugar content), it was no doubt contributing to his insomnia.*

> Coffee, tea, chocolate, many soft drinks (particularly colas and "energy drinks"), and even some medications contain caffeine.

## Cigarettes

How is it that many smokers say that they find smoking relaxing when the nicotine in cigarettes is a drug that, like caffeine, is a stimulant? The answer lies in the association many smokers make between lighting up a cigarette and relaxation. It is a psychological link which may make smoking appear to be an aid to sleep. Yet we know that, due to its stimulating effects, smoking is much more likely to disrupt sleep. Heavy smokers will also find their sleep is affected because each night they will be suffering withdrawal symptoms. If you typically smoke a cigarette (or more) every waking hour, then your body gets used to this injection of nicotine and finds it difficult to go without its regular dose of nicotine for a prolonged stretch of seven or eight hours. If your body is undergoing withdrawal symptoms each night, you can't expect to sleep peacefully and without disturbance.

Not only are smoking and nicotine detrimental to your health, smoking specifically affects breathing, and breathing problems commonly contribute to sleep problems. These factors all point to the potentially problematic effects of smoking on your sleep. Although this is a guide to better sleep and not a program particularly aimed at smoking cessation, it is suggested that if you desire good sleep you should aim towards an overall, healthy lifestyle. As such, quitting, or at least reducing, the number of cigarettes you smoke, may well be worth trying. Once again, however, this can be difficult to do on your own. You may want to consult your local doctor or find a specialist service or program dedicated to helping people achieve this goal.

## On a positive note

So far, this section has focused on food and drink that disrupt sleep. There are also drinks that can induce good sleep:

- Although they do not work for everyone, certain herbal teas have a relaxing effect and, therefore, improve sleep. The best known for their sedative properties are valerian and chamomile.
- A cup of warm milk at night has long been recommended by mothers and grandmothers and there is scientific support for this recommendation. Milk contains an amino acid known as L-tryptophan, which is associated with serotonin, a naturally occurring drug in the brain. There are indications

that milk increases serotonin, which, in turn, enhances sleep.

Whether a warm mug of milk or herbal tea contains sleep-inducing properties or not is actually not that important. What is probably most significant is that a nice, warm, non-alcoholic, non-caffeinated drink taken before retiring for the night can be very relaxing. It is this sense of relaxation that is more likely to help with sleep.

So eat well and in moderation, cut back or consider eliminating altogether the sleeping potions, the alcohol, the caffeine and the nicotine, curl up with a warm mug of milk or herbal tea at bedtime, and drift off to a better sleep!

# Exercise and be active

## The relationship between exercise and sleep

Sleep and exercise are as different as night and day, yet they are linked to one another. Without adequate sleep, you won't get far with your physical exertions; and, as we shall see, without sufficient regular exercise, your sleep suffers. So the two—sleep and exercise—are inextricably linked, though they are at opposite ends of a hypothetical activity spectrum.

Sleep involves mental and physical relaxation, the minimization of arousal so as to reach a state of calm and tranquillity. Exercise involves physical and physiological arousal, intentional effort and working your body hard, usually in fairly rapid movements. Sleep involves little or no movement (not conscious or intentional movement, at any rate). Despite their differences, regular exercise is an essential part of the Good Sleep Program, just as it should be part of a healthy lifestyle. To reiterate: one of the central tenets of *The Good Sleep Guide* is that healthy sleep is associated with healthy living. As we saw in the previous chapter, a healthy diet will help you to live, function, and feel better. A healthy exercise program can consolidate and improve upon these results.

 Regular exercise is an essential part of the Good Sleep Program.

Regular exercise has been found to enhance a sense of well being (including the positive psychological state of feeling in a good mood) and to be associated with higher levels of energy and motivation. Increasingly, the antidepressant benefits of exercise are being recognized, and in recent years psychological programs aimed at treating depression and anxiety have increasingly included exercise for the benefits it bestows. Most importantly, regular exercise is associated with better sleep.

## Activity versus exercise

But what is "regular exercise" and how does it differ from "activity?" Can you still keep fit and healthy without having to run a marathon or compete at the highest level?

The good news is that you do not have to work as hard as an elite athlete in training to derive the benefits of regular exercise. In fact, the athlete's level of activity is not appropriate or necessary for most of us. You can derive benefits from a generally active lifestyle without exercising at a level that involves physical discomfort. And let's admit it, although we should all keep active, the reality is that many of us do not enjoy strenuous activity.

General activity is particularly important for people who have a sedentary lifestyle or a desk-bound job. Rapidly increasing numbers of us spend most, if not all, of our days at a desk in front of a computer screen, then spend most of our evenings relaxing in front of the TV, reading, listening to music, on the phone, surfing the Net or chatting. Furthermore, many of us spend our working lives in air-conditioned buildings with only rare (and usually brief) excursions away from the desk and with little, if any, exposure to the normal daily changes in light and temperature.

If you fall into this group of people who do not achieve the necessary and appropriate levels of activity (let alone exercise!) in their normal daily routines, you will have to make that extra effort to reach physical activity levels that will ensure you gain the benefits of a healthy, active lifestyle.

In the sections that follow, I will briefly discuss what is involved in activity and exercise (specific and planned efforts to improve fitness and/or strength) and how you can achieve a reasonable level that should help you to be healthier and, consequently, sleep better.

# A healthy, active lifestyle

Before we discuss focused and regular exercise, let's explore the many ways we can keep generally active. A wealth of scientific research findings indicate that even without regular exercise, people who keep relatively active are healthier and less likely to experience cardiac and other associated health problems. In short, people who keep active are more likely to live longer.

Keeping active also contributes to a better quality of life. Just think about it, people who are more active are more able and likely to engage in a range of activities and are therefore more likely to be challenged and satisfied. Not surprisingly, people who are active are happier and more confident individuals than their inactive, sedentary counterparts.

> Here are some places you will find happiness: the gym, the swimming pool, the footpath or bicycle path.

There are numerous ways for you to keep active and the number of options is only limited by your imagination. Keeping active can be as simple as walking to the local shops for bread and milk rather than driving. Keeping active can mean going to the local park with your partner and/or your children, or your dog, rather than sitting at home watching TV. Keeping active frequently means driving less and walking more.

Catching public transport more often will lead to you being more active. Walking to the bus stop or train station is likely to require more activity than sitting in your car. If you want to go for a drive, by all means do so, but incorporate into your outing a stop for a walk, or a swim, or a stroll down the shopping strip, or a play on the swings.

Anything that requires some exertion and movement qualifies as activity. Even gentle activities like wandering around a gallery or a museum count because they require you to be up and on your feet, not slouched in a beanbag. But, sorry, it is not enough to simply move your channel-changing trigger finger! Nor is leaning forward every five minutes to pass around the bowl of salted nuts!

You can even become more active while you are at work. Rather than catching the lift, take the opportunity to get some exercise walking up and down the stairs. Rather than calling or emailing your colleague down the hall, or in another office, get up and walk over to them. Go for a short walk at lunch. Get out of the office and away from the fluorescent lights and airconditioning, and out into the fresh air and natural light. All of these things help you to achieve a healthier, more active lifestyle.

 Walk up or down the stairs instead of taking the lift. If you must take an escalator, don't glide—stride!

Some of these suggestions might seem very small, almost insignificant steps, but small things add up to bigger things. Every drop in the ocean of activity can help. Sometimes it is the smallest things that can make the most difference.

*When I began to discuss these ideas with Paul he was having difficulty keeping a straight face. Paul is a busy stockbroker who works long hours (at least twelve a day); he could barely find time to come and see me, let alone take time away from his desk for a lunch break. Not surprisingly, Paul was desperate. He was so disheartened by not sleeping well that he agreed to try some small changes. We agreed to start small, so as not to overly disrupt his busy schedule. He agreed to take at least half an hour for lunch and try to get out of his office. Initially, he did not believe it would achieve anything, but he was desperate, so decided to give it a go.*

*What happened was remarkable. Taking a very short lunchbreak made an enormous difference. Paul reported that he felt as though a weight had been lifted from his shoulders. He told me that taking a break in the middle of the day made his afternoons much easier. Rather than feeling as though he could barely make it through the day, he said that the break refreshed him. He felt revitalized and re-energized, significantly more relaxed and, therefore, better able to cope with the remainder of the day and the evening.*

*Moreover, this effect snowballed. Because he was feeling refreshed after lunch, Paul discovered he was more productive and his interactions with his colleagues were more pleasant.*

*Also he found that he was feeling much less stressed when he returned home to his wife and children. He had more patience and tolerance with them (and they noticed). They told him that they appreciated his improved mood, which made him feel even better. As a result of these improvements in himself, at work and at home, Paul resolved to continue doing what had helped—at least three to four times each week he went for short walks at lunchtime.*

 Instead of shouting to someone in a nearby room, or using the office intercom, take the opportunity to get up and stretch your legs. Exercise your muscles, not your vocal chords.

You too may be surprised to find that a few minutes of light activity here and there can make such a difference. Like Paul, you too will find that there is a lot to gain, so go on and give it a try! Look for opportunities to go for a short walk. Take opportunities to be active. Make a point of getting up and walking away from your desk. It is really so simple: just move about and you will feel (and those around you will begin to notice) the benefits.

## Regular exercise

As well as increasing your levels of general activity, you should try to engage in at least thirty minutes or more of vigorous, aerobic exercise, at least three to four times each week. That means *you*. (Yes, and me too; in fact, it means all of us.) Everyone should engage in some form of regular exercise.

By "regular exercise" I mean activity that is both qualitatively and quantitatively more than the general activity discussed above. Regular exercise is not just walking to the bus stop, or walking up the stairs. It is real exercise.

 Aim to get 30 minutes of aerobic exercise every other day.

*Like many people, Sonia complained, "I don't have time for sport." She had enjoyed sport at school, and apparently had been relatively good at it, but since leaving school her focus had been on her studies and then on her career. Although she knew that exercise was recommended for good health and for good sleep, she simply could not imagine herself fitting any regular form of exercise into her already over-busy routine.*

What Sonia did not realize, however, is that there are many ways you can exercise. Again, the number of options is only limited by your imagination. Traditionally, exercise takes the form of jogging or going to an organized exercise class (such as aerobics) in a gym. However, because exercise can be any form of activity that is at least moderately strenuous, it can take the form of walking with a friend or with the dog (at a reasonable pace), playing sports such as tennis or squash, surfing, swimming, throwing a ball in the park, riding a bike or rollerblading. In fact, exercise can be anything that gets your body moving energetically and, ideally, gets your heart pumping, for a useful period of time.

## HOW MUCH ACTIVITY AND EXERCISE IS ENOUGH?

It is generally recommended that you do the equivalent of at least thirty minutes of walking every day to fulfill your activity quota. This thirty minutes need not be all at the same time, but, if you can fit in several short walks throughout the course of your day, you can gain physically and improve your overall health, without even realizing it.

To review, you could try walking to the bus stop or to the train station. Better still, walk to work or get off public transport one stop early and walk the rest of the way. Walk up and down the stairs (or escalator) rather than catching the lift. Take a short stroll during your lunchbreak and generally try to take advantage of any opportunities you can to move about as much as possible. If you can accumulate approximately thirty minutes of this type of general activity daily, then you are providing yourself with the opportunity to be healthier (and, of course, to sleep better).

And, be assured, you will be healthier. Medical research suggests that people who engage in as little as thirty minutes of gentle activity on a regular, daily basis are significantly less likely to develop health problems over the course of their lives. Notably, these people are much less likely to develop cardiac (heart) and respiratory (breathing) problems. And don't forget: good health is associated with good sleep.

 Take out medical insurance: walk for 30 minutes every day.

Above and beyond fulfilling your activity quota, you should try to get at least three to four sessions of vigorous exercise every week. Many people would recommend that this is the minimum and that more would be helpful. It depends, however, on you and your lifestyle. Exercising three to four times each week will help. But exercising five or six times will help even more and you'll feel the benefits sooner. Three to four sessions are certainly worthwhile, so if this is all you can fit into a busy schedule, that is fine. The important thing is to start somewhere and get into a regular routine.

## WHAT QUALIFIES AS EXERCISE?

Running, jogging, rapid walking, swimming, bicycling or anything else that involves you in regular strenuous exercise will contribute to better health and therefore to better sleep. Regular exercise is associated with weight control which is something for troubled sleepers to consider since being overweight can increase your chances of respiratory and other medical problems that can affect your sleep.

## A NOTE OF CAUTION

As with many of the suggestions in this guide, if you have any reasons to be concerned about exercising, consult your doctor first. In particular, talk to your doctor before beginning a new exercise program if:

- you have any history of heart or respiratory problems, or if anyone in your family has
- you are significantly overweight
- you have any other relevant health problems.

Your doctor will be able to advise you whether it is safe for you to proceed with an exercise program. It probably will be, because, even if you have one of these problems, exercise is frequently recommended as a way of improving your health. But there may be specific precautions you need to take and your doctor will be able to recommend how best to conduct your new exercise regime. Once you have talked to your doctor and been given the go-ahead, begin slowly and gradually so as to minimize any risk of injury. If you have never seriously engaged in a regular exercise program before, then it might be worth seeking the advice of an appropriate professional, such as a physiotherapist or a personal trainer (or one of the staff at your local gym or health club).

# Motivation to keep it up

Invariably, when I come to discuss this part of the program with my patients they nod in agreement, and they say things like "Yes, yes . . . I know I really need to exercise more. Yes,

I'll start tomorrow." We all know we *should* exercise regularly. Even those of us who do engage in some form of regular activity and exercise realize we could benefit more if we exercized more.

And most people are aware that the benefits are not just physical, but that there are psychological benefits as well. Frequently people tell me that they feel better when they are exercising. Many exercise solely for the stress-relieving benefits; gyms are full of people "letting off steam," running off their daily hassles, "working out" their problems and their worries. Some of them even realize that regular exercise is also associated with improved sleep.

It is clear and generally known that exercise is:

- simple
- accessible
- not necessarily expensive (discounting shoe leather!)
- physically and psychologically beneficial
- a must for everyone who wants to live a long and healthy life.

So it is astonishing that there are people who do not exercise. But then again knowing human nature . . . it is one thing *to know* something is good for you and quite another thing *to act* on that knowledge.

The most frequently cited reason for not exercising is a lack of time: "I'm too busy. I just don't have the time." I'm frequently told by the people who come to see me that they work long hours, have to do the household chores, have children and pets and maybe aging parents to care for, as well as friends to see, not to mention cars to wash, houses to renovate, and lawns to mow!

These are all very compelling reasons and who is to deny that these tasks really do need to be done? But what I can't avoid hearing when I'm told "I don't have the time" is that other message: "I would rather spend my time doing other things. I have other priorities. I choose to spend my time doing these other activities rather than exercising." And since in the short term there are relatively few negative consequences to not exercising, regular exercise tends not to gain priority status for most busy people focused on "getting through the day."

The point is you have a choice. Rather than considering whether or not you are prepared to make sleep a priority, we are now talking about whether or not you are prepared to class exercise among your priorities. Conveniently, doing so is linked with making sleep a priority, because, as we now know, exercise enables improved sleep.

 Need more time? It's simple: sleep more and get your daily exercise. You'll have more energy, get more done in less time, and so make time for other things.

People who do make sleep a priority tend to be able to find time to do other new things as well—such as making exercise a priority. How can this be? How is it possible that people who have made sleep and exercise priorities in their lives actually find they have *more* time to do other things?

They don't actually have more time, of course (there are, after all, only 24 hours in a day), but these sleep-and-exercise-prioritizing people now find that they have more energy and feel better. Having more energy allows them to get more done. So long as you organize your time sensibly, you will have more energy and desire to do more.

## AN EXERCISE TO HELP YOU GAIN MOTIVATION TO EXERCISE

If you are still struggling to motivate yourself to start, or to maintain, an exercise program, try this.

Take a sheet of paper and draw a line down the centre. On the top left-hand side, write and underline "Problems associated with inactivity and not exercising." On the top right-hand side, write and underline "Benefits associated with keeping active and exercising regularly."

Now list as many things as you can think of under each heading. If you can think of only a few things, then talk to a family member or a friend and see if they can generate some more ideas. Hopefully, after you have thought about it for a while and, if necessary, discussed it with someone else, you will have a long list. You should be able to think of lots of reasons why inactivity is not good for you. Further, you should be able to think of lots of reasons why activity and exercise are good for you. If you can't generate a long list, then you are unlikely to exercise regularly and you probably need to talk to someone further about this issue. Try to keep the list somewhere you can see it often and review it regularly. This list should provide the motivation you need to start or continue some form of exercise program.

## BEGIN YOUR EXERCISE PROGRAM SLOWLY AND GRADUALLY

Many people get all fired up, charge in to the gym and work out hectically for a few days, or maybe a few weeks, and then crash in a heap. Their muscles quickly become sore, their joints ache, they may incur injuries—in short, they overdo it. They stop for a few weeks to recover and then, likely as not, give up. Obviously, this approach defeats the purpose, is a waste of time (and possibly of money), punishes your body, and is bad for your morale.

So beware of falling into this trap. The only form of effective exercise is regular and sustained over a prolonged period of time. One or two weeks' worth achieves little. One or two months' worth achieves only a little more. To really experience the benefits of exercise, physically and psychologically, it needs to become a regular part of your lifestyle. Exercise needs to become something you do on a regular basis, just like brushing your teeth or showering.

## SET A CONVENIENT TIME TO EXERCISE

You need to decide what time of day suits you best to exercise. It needs to fit around your other commitments. There is no point trying to walk or jog at 7.30 every morning if this is a hectic time of the day when you need to prepare yourself for work, iron a school play costume, pack the lunches, feed the cat, track down that missing soccer jersey, lock up the house, and drive the children to school!

## FIND A FORM OF EXERCISE THAT SUITS YOU

For exercise to become part of your lifestyle, you need to find something you will be happy doing regularly and repeatedly. You may get a kick out of belonging to a gym, being with others and having all the staff and equipment available for you—or you may detest the idea and prefer to run a mile (that's a form of exercise) to avoid a room of bouncing, perspiring aerobic jazzercizers and sweating, steroid-pumped-up musclemen heaving weights! You can get extremely fit and healthy without going in the vicinity of a gym. Anyone for tennis? Or if you can easily get to the beach or a pool, you could swim. Have you got a dog or child (or grandchild) in a pusher you could take for walks? Perhaps you could bicycle or jog.

## VARY YOUR ACTIVITIES

Anything that is done over and over can become boring, even if it is something you enjoy. If it bores you, you are more likely to neglect it and eventually abandon it altogether. If your exercise regime begins to become rather monotonous, you will need to quickly find other forms of exercise that will engage your interest. Don't delay finding a substitute, because physical gains from exercising can be lost very quickly. That is why it is so important to exercise regularly, so that you keep experiencing the benefits.

Variety is the spice of life, so be prepared to vary your exercise: this can be the key to maintaining an exercise program in the long term. To avoid boredom, exercise in different ways. In summer, get out and walk or jog or swim. In winter, find a heated pool or a gym that you like. In summer, play tennis or soccer. In winter, try indoor sports such as squash or basketball.

## MAKE IT FUN

Exercise should not be a torture. In fact, it is crucial to ensure it is fun. Exercise can be made more enjoyable by listening to your favorite music on a portable stereo player. Exercise and activity can be more enjoyable if you do it with someone you like. Find a friend who might be interested in walking or running with you regularly. Better still, find a group of friends who can all join in some activity together. This can lead to your exercise becoming a social outing, making it all the more rewarding.

## KEEP RECORDS

Keeping records is also helpful so that you can monitor your progress and won't forget what you have achieved. At the end of a long day when you are tired and not feeling like you want to exercise, it is too easy to focus on how hard it all is and how you feel you are not really getting anywhere. Having a written record, however, can remind you that you are progressing and that you really are getting somewhere. Seeing this in black and white can be very motivating. Or you may want to plot your performance on a graph to offer you more inspiration and a sense of accomplishment.

## REWARD YOURSELF

It is important to reward yourself when you exercise, as this can drastically improve your chances of keeping up with your exercise program. Especially in the early stages, plan what you want to have accomplished. Planning also helps you to avoid the I'll-wait-and-see-how-I-feel phenomenon which usually turns into the I'll-wait-forever-and-ever-or-until-a-magic-wand-taps-me-on-the-shoulder problem.

So, right now set yourself a reasonable goal of a certain number of times (say four) per week that you will exercise for at least thirty minutes. Commit to maintaining that routine for, say, a fortnight and then be sure, if you have achieved this goal, that you give yourself a reward.

When you've achieved your specific goals or land-marks, give yourself a pat on the back. You might also like to buy yourself a small present. Or simply wait until you have achieved a goal before buying yourself that new book or CD that you have been wanting. This sounds simple, maybe even "childish," but it is an extremely effective strategy. By finding a way of rewarding yourself that you are comfortable with, you will be more likely to continue with your exercise program. The more you keep to your exercise program, the more likely you are to be healthy. If you are healthy, you are more likely to sleep well.

# CHAPTER 5

# Learn to relax

## Tension and stress

*When Paul came for his first assessment he appeared perfectly normal—apart from being somewhat tired and irritable.*

*These are common symptoms of persistent insomnia. So too is tension (muscular tightness), and as Paul sat through the initial interview it was clear that he was not comfortable in his chair. When asked, he said he'd never had any back or neck injuries but did report frequently experiencing aches and pains, especially in his shoulders and neck, and that he was prone to headaches. He said that he felt tight and tense and his muscles*

*almost always felt stiff. Paul was describing the classic*
*symptoms of tension.*

*When Sonia first came for an assessment she did not display any*
*of the signs of physical tension that I had observed in Paul, but*
*she certainly did appear to be tense or stressed in a slightly*
*different way. Rather than having raised shoulders and a*
*clenched jaw, as Paul did, Sonia's stress was reflected in her*
*tapping feet and busy fingers. It was as though she could not sit*
*still and she constantly checked her watch to monitor the time.*
*When I commented on this, and asked whether she was*
*concerned about something, she stated that she had a lot to do*
*at work and really should be getting back there. She was very*
*concerned about being late back to her desk. After assuring*
*her that I would keep track of the clock and make sure that we*
*finished on time, she continued nervously checking her watch*
*and made passing reference to all the tasks waiting for her*
*at the office.*

*She had come to see me because she was not sleeping and*
*was now experiencing a range of problems secondary to her*
*sleep problem, yet she could not take the undivided time*
*to talk to me about her sleeping problems without being*
*constantly distracted by the pressures of her life.*

These two case studies reflect how *tension* and *stress* are
related, but different. Although often used synonymously,
the two terms will be used in this guide to denote slightly
different problems:

- "Tension" will be used to refer to the more *physical* aspects of the problem, most notably, tight muscles. Muscles can be tensed intentionally, such as when we flex the muscles in our forearm in order to open a new jar of jam, or they can become tense without conscious effort, such as when we are exposed to long-term stress.

- On the other hand, "stress" is used here to denote an essentially *emotional* problem. It is related to worry and anxiety. Although usually associated with a negative state, "stress" is derived from the Greek words: *eustress* and *dystress*. *Eustress* was "good stress," or stress that motivated you to perform better (such as the excitement a dancer, musician or athlete experiences just before going out to perform). In contrast, *dystress* (or distress) referred to "bad stress" that impeded or disrupted performance (such as being so agitated that you forget your lines or freeze in the midst of an exam). These days, stress is most often used in this negative sense.

- Tension refers to the physical aspects of the problem (e.g. tight muscles).
- Stress refers to the emotional problem (e.g. worry and anxiety).

Tension and stress frequently occur together: one tends to lead to and exacerbate the other, as we all know. Scientific research has found a link between worry and muscle tension. Clinical experience also suggests that the two can often become entwined in a vicious circle. The more stress you feel emotionally, the more your muscles tense. The increase in muscular tension adds to the level of stress. This can continue indefinitely, unless something is done to stop it.

Prolonged physical tension is uncomfortable, even painful, which contributes to stress as the sufferer begins to worry about how long they will have to endure the discomfort and what they can do about it. Similarly, long-term emotional stress takes its toll on the body and can lead to muscles becoming tense.

## How relaxation can help

Although not the miracle cure some people profess it to be, relaxation is one of the most important components of any sleep program. In fact, like exercise and a sensible diet, regular relaxation is an important component in any healthy lifestyle program. Most importantly, relaxation can make it easier for you to get to sleep and increase your chances of staying asleep. Being relaxed can also improve the quality of your sleep.

Relaxation assists with sleep because it tackles two of the enemies of sleep: tension and stress. Clearly, if these two problems are not sufficiently addressed, they can significantly contribute to delayed sleep onset and disrupted sleep throughout the night. Learning how to relax can help to break the vicious circle referred to above. Relaxation significantly reduces muscle tension, and it helps to control, even eliminate, worrying thoughts. Relaxation contributes to an enhanced sense of well being and to better psychological health, which, in turn, can assist most people to get better sleep.

## What is relaxation?

For some people, relaxation is soaking in a hot bath with some enjoyable music playing in the background. For others, it is working towards a meditative state in which heightened levels of consciousness are the goal. Although many of the people I see are seeking some form of relaxation, or are trying to learn how to achieve more effective relaxation more often, they are not all seeking the same outcome.

> Paul, for example, wanted to feel looser and wanted the tightness in his muscles to ease. Sonia, on the other hand, after being helped to understand her problems better, wanted to be able to shut down her mind for a while and experience some peace from intrusive, demanding and racing thoughts.

Relaxation can be a few minutes of tranquil thought, a deep breath to help you get through a difficult situation, or an altered state of consciousness when striving for spiritual enlightenment.

Meditation that seeks to achieve a purer level of consciousness, a greater level of awareness, and a higher self will not be covered in this guide. Similar to prayer, meditation has many benefits that have been documented and acknowledged. However, significant amounts of time must be devoted to master the complexities of this art.

Relaxation, as will be discussed here, although similar in some ways to meditation, can be achieved much more quickly and easily to reduce tension and stress. Its aim is to help you cope with your daily stresses and with sources of tension. Most importantly, the relaxation techniques described in this guide are primarily aimed to help you to sleep better. To master the skill of relaxation you will need to practice for a few minutes, several times each day. Once you have learned how to relax, you'll find that you feel less stressed, less tense, more calm and able to sleep better.

## How to relax

If you visit the self-help section of your nearest bookshop to see how many relaxation, meditation or stress-management books are available, you will appreciate that there is more than one way to relax. We are all different and the ways we relax differ from person to person. No one strategy or approach to relaxation will work for every person.

The aim of this chapter, therefore, is to introduce you to a few of the more commonly used and effective relaxation strategies.

## WHICH STRATEGY WILL WORK FOR YOU?

I suggest you try several strategies and then decide which one works best for you. Remember that there is no right or wrong way to relax; it is just a matter of finding *your* method of relaxation and then using it every day.

To begin, let's try two of the most commonly used relaxation strategies recommended by psychologists and psychiatrists. Although they are very simple, they are also very effective methods of relaxation. They have the additional benefit of being able to be applied almost anywhere and at any time.

These two strategies form the basis of other forms of relaxation, such as meditation and self-hypnosis. They can be used together, or on their own:

- "Relaxation Strategy 1: Relax your mind" focuses on dealing with stress. If your main problem is worry, stress, frustration or anxiety, then you should definitely try this (you should also read Chapter 8 on healthy thinking).

- "Relaxation Strategy 2: Relax your body" focuses on reducing tension. If you are troubled by tension (including constant aches and pains), then this strategy may be of more benefit to you (and you may want to consider reviewing Chapter 4 on exercise and activity).

## RELAXATION STRATEGY 1: RELAX YOUR MIND

The idea of this strategy is to focus your mind on something simple and relaxing. I don't recommend that you try to *clear* your mind since most people find this very difficult or impossible. I don't think it is necessary to *empty* your mind of all thoughts in order to relax. This is exceptionally difficult to do and for many unachievable. Rather, the idea is to find a simple and calming word or phrase, or maybe a relaxing and pleasant image on which to focus. The more you focus on this word or image, the less likely you are to have worrying and stressful thoughts.

So remember, the idea is not necessarily to clear your mind, but rather to focus as much as possible on one simple, calming thing.

The first step is to be seated upright in a firm but comfortable chair and to breathe slowly and evenly. Regular breathing is an integral part of all forms of relaxation and its importance cannot be underestimated. At the same time, however, it is important to avoid one of the more common pitfalls of relaxation that stems from a common belief that you need to breathe "deeply" in order to relax. This is not necessarily true. In fact, breathing too deeply can lead to hyperventilation, which can produce symptoms similar to anxiety (such as increased heart rate, dizziness and sweating), thereby making it very difficult to relax.

> The first step to relaxation is breathing in a slow, smooth, regular fashion.

Instead, I always recommend that people try to breathe slowly and evenly, rather than deeply. Your body will know how deeply it needs to breathe. It will do this automatically. What you need to do is let your body do its job and try not to interfere or apply force.

So focus on breathing at a nice, slow pace, letting each breath come and go, as it wants to. If you can allow your body to breathe nice and slowly, and if you can achieve this regularly, you will have come a long way towards relaxation already.

In addition, it is important to *focus your mind* and to let go of the mental stress you are experiencing. Probably the easiest way to do this is to focus on a simple word (which serves the function of the mantra of meditation). For many people the word "relax" is easy and helpful to use. Just saying it can do the trick of setting you at ease. To stay focused, use your breathing to help you to time your repetition of the word "relax." Since there are two stages to breathing (the inspiration and the expiration), it can be helpful to have another word to say as well as "relax." To keep it simple, I usually recommend the word "in."

So putting all of this together, all you need to do is to allow your body to settle into a nice steady pattern of breathing—breathing slowly and evenly, not necessarily deeply—and repeat the two simple words "in" (as you breathe in) and "relax" (as you breathe out). There is no need to say these words out loud, just say them quietly to yourself, over and over again in the back of your mind. Say "in" as you breathe in, and "relax" as you breathe out. Continue this simple and relaxing pattern for as long as you can or for as long as you like (between five and ten minutes).

And that's all there is to it! Because it is straightforward and, compared to some other strategies, quick and easy to use, it can (once you practice enough and become proficient in it) be used anywhere and any time. This simple and easy-to-learn strategy has changed many lives and has helped many people to feel more relaxed and to sleep better.

## RELAXATION STRATEGY 2: RELAX YOUR BODY

Whereas the first strategy is mostly aimed at stress and worry, this second strategy is more focused on trying to release the physical tension that can build up in your muscles. Accomplishing this can reduce the intensity of aches and pains, thereby helping you to feel more comfortable, and, consequently, improving your sleep.

Reducing tension can also lead to a number of other benefits, such as increased energy. If you walk around tense all day, you are, unintentionally, wasting considerable amounts of energy that can cause unnecessary tiredness. By conserving your energy rather than wasting it on useless tension, you can direct it towards more worthwhile endeavors.

The first step of this strategy is to make yourself comfortable. Ideally, the best position is to be sitting in a comfortable chair. Although lying down may seem to be the most comfortable position, the sitting position is preferred because you need to develop a strategy that can be applied in a whole range of situations (not just when you are going to bed). In many circumstances it is not possible to lie down when you get stressed or when you feel tense.

With this in mind, make yourself comfortable, and begin to breathe slowly in the same way as was described for Relaxation Strategy 1. Just breathe in and out, nice and slowly, and let your body determine its own, natural pace. Once you have settled into a steady rhythm, *try to relax all of your muscles*. Very few people can do this all at once, so this form of relaxation (commonly referred to as "progressive muscle relaxation") involves two steps:

1   Gently tense your muscles, one group at a time.

2   Then relax different groups of muscles one at a time, rather than trying to relax them all in one go.

The muscles in your body can be divided into groups. Sixteen different muscle groups have been identified, but I usually recommend working on the following five:

1   head and face

2   neck and shoulders

3   arms and hands

4   abdomen, body and back

5   legs and feet.

The most common sites of muscle tension are the neck and shoulders, jaw and/or your temples (the sides of your head, near your eyes). This strategy can be used on any or all of these locations.

So, pulling the various components of Relaxation Strategy 2 together, simply start by breathing slowly, and then begin to concentrate on a particular body part or muscle group. If you intend to try relaxing more than one of the muscle groups listed above, it is generally recommended that you start at the top with the head and face, and slowly work your way down through your body, ending with your feet.

Gently tense the relevant muscles for a few seconds as you breathe in. Don't do this so hard that it hurts, but tighten the muscles just hard enough to begin to notice the tension. Tensing your muscles as you breathe in, hold the tension for a few seconds, continuing to breathe slowly in and out. Then, after a few breaths, let the tension go as you breathe out. Continue this for several minutes, focusing on each muscle group, and work your way down your body.

That's all there is to it! As with the first strategy, this is easy to learn and the gains can be considerable within a relatively short period of time. This tried-and-tested strategy can help you to feel substantially better, physically and mentally, in a matter of days or weeks.

## Maximizing the gains from relaxation

To get the most out of relaxation you will need to devote some time to making it work for you. With both of these strategies, and in fact with any form of relaxation, one of the most important determinants of how much you will benefit will be how often you practice. Relaxation is a skill and, like any other skill, the more you practice the better you will get at it. Ideally, you should practice several (e.g. four or five) times each day. Each session need only be for five to ten minutes, which if added up comes to less than an hour a day.

Regular practice is important to enable you to master the skill, but it is important for another reason. It is highly unlikely that the stress and/or tension that is disrupting your sleep suddenly appears when you lie down in your bed at night. It is more likely that the stress and tension build up gradually throughout the day as you face the myriad little difficulties (at work, at home, at the shops, in traffic). As such, practicing relaxation regularly can reduce this build-up and defuse or release the total amount of stress or tension that you will be carrying with you to bed. Notably, these strategies will also help you to deal with stress throughout the day. They are not just useful for sleep, but are an integral part of stress management.

This is why, as noted above, it is important to practice these relaxation techniques in a range of situations—not just at home, lying in your bed. I usually recommend that people try to apply these strategies wherever and whenever they can. This can be done by stopping everything and having a good break, or, alternatively, once you have mastered the skills, by practicing one of the relaxation strategies while you are doing something else: waiting on the phone; waiting for (or riding on) public transport; standing in a queue, or anywhere. Although it can help to close your eyes while trying to relax (this minimizes the chances of distraction), both of these strategies can work just as well with your eyes open. Not surprisingly, some of you may not want to close your eyes if trying to relax in public!

So practice often and practice anywhere. Since some

people find effective relaxation more difficult to achieve, don't necessarily expect these strategies to work immediately. To relax effectively, you will probably need to work at it, but with time and practice you will master the technique and feel the considerable benefits.

## Overcoming common problems

The two relaxation strategies described above are easy to do and most readers should benefit within a relatively short period of time. However, for those people who find they are experiencing difficulty, this section reviews some of the more common problems you may encounter when trying to relax, along with some suggestions for overcoming these problems and for allowing the relaxation strategies to help you manage stress, tension and poor sleep.

In my experience, probably the most common problem has to do with other, distracting, non-relaxing thoughts disrupting your relaxation sessions. If worrying or intrusive thoughts come into your mind, it can be difficult to achieve a calm and relaxed state. If this is your problem, be reassured that you are not alone. Most people just starting to learn the art of relaxation have this problem.

Strange as this may sound, it is important that you do not try to fight distracting, intrusive thoughts. Don't let them make you angry or frustrated. Fighting these sorts of interruptive thoughts tends to make them fight back, and then they become even more difficult to overcome.

Instead, if you find yourself distracted by other thoughts, ask yourself this question. Am I relaxed? If you are relaxed, despite your thoughts wandering off onto something else, then fine. Remember that the aim is to relax and different people relax in different ways. For some, letting their minds wander can be the best way to do it. But if the answer is no, and you find that you are worrying or becoming stressed or tense, then gently bring your attention back to your breathing and to those two simple words: "in" and "relax." You may need to do this sort of refocusing several times when you are starting to learn to relax. But, as you practice more you will get more proficient, and, as you get better, you will find that you can maintain your focus for longer periods of time without becoming distracted.

If you are continually distracted by a serious worry or by a significant problem, then it might be best to take what steps you can to remove the source of the worries. In this case, I suggest you refer to Chapter 7 for advice on problem solving and time management and/or Chapter 8 for suggestions on how to deal with worry and negative, ruminating thoughts. Although there are many situations where relaxation can be extremely helpful, there are some where you simply need to act. In this case, it might be difficult to properly relax until you have tackled the problem.

It is crucial that you don't give up early on. Give yourself at least four to six weeks of regular practice. It can take this long to master any skill and it can take this long to reverse some of the old, unhelpful habits that have been causing your stress and tension. Also, don't give up on an individual session until you have tried for at least a few minutes. If you are using relaxation to try to go to sleep, don't ever give up, even if you don't go to sleep. Think to yourself that you have a choice. You can lie in bed awake and stressed. Or you can lie in bed awake, but relaxed. Lying in bed relaxed is far better than lying in bed tense and frustrated. Lying in bed relaxed can be very restorative. In fact, it can be almost as good as sleeping. Even if you are following the guidelines set out in Chapter 6 for sleep restriction or stimulus control (which may entail getting out of bed at times during the night), it is still important to try to stay as relaxed as you can.

Finally, some people experience problems because they expect too much of relaxation. This can cause them to feel disappointed if their (possibly unrealistic) expectations are not met. Remember the distinction we made between relaxation and meditation? If you are seeking a means to a higher state of consciousness, relaxation is quite likely not the vehicle that's going to do it for you. Expecting relaxation to fulfill some spiritual need or to transform your life is unrealistic. (Of course, by enabling you to sleep and overcome your tiredness, relaxation will change your life for the better.) For relaxation to be most effective, it is critical that your expectations of it are realistic. The two forms of relaxation suggested can help you to reduce stress and tension, and to sleep better.

# Other useful strategies

In the first instance, I usually encourage people to try the two relatively simple and easy-to-learn relaxation methods I've already mentioned, and to persevere with them for several weeks before trying other strategies.

However, there are a number of variations on these two strategies which some people might find more helpful. Once you've given the first two strategies a try and, ideally, mastered at least one of them, you may wish to consider the modified versions described below and add them to, or combine them with, the two basic forms.

## PLEASANT IMAGERY RELAXATION

One of the most common variations on the simple "in and relax" method is generally referred to as "pleasant imagery" relaxation. As the name suggests, it involves imagining something pleasant and, of course, relaxing. Essentially, it involves starting off in the same way as that described for Relaxation Strategy 1, but, rather than focusing exclusively on the two words "in" and "relax," the emphasis is more on focusing on a pleasant scene or situation. The good thing about this method is that it can be any image, scene or situation you like, as long as it is calming and relaxing. Consider these examples:

a) Imagine that you are reclining in a hammock, on an idyllic desert island, on a perfect summer's day.

It is warm, but not too hot. There is a pleasant breeze gently blowing. The sky is beautifully blue. The water is crystal clear and is quietly lapping against the clean, white sand of the beach. There are coconut palms rustling in the breeze and gulls gliding through the air. All is calm. All is peaceful. You are perfectly content and happy, wanting nothing, needing nothing. You are relaxed.

b) Imagine that you are in a beautifully restored, old timber hut in the midst of an untouched forested wilderness. Outside it is cool and fresh. There is a sprinkling of snow on the ground and on the branches of the tall trees. After returning refreshed and invigorated from an energetic walk, you have just finished a delicious and nourishing meal. You are now seated in a comfortable armchair in front of a blazing log fire. It is comfortably warm. You are physically tired and mentally relaxed. Everything around you is peaceful and calm. There is quiet music playing in the background. It is just the right sort of music for the setting. You are content. You are relaxed.

You may wish to use either of these examples, or create your own ideal scene (revisit a pleasant memory, borrow a scene from a film or a book, or tailor-make your own relaxation landscape). It can be whatever you like, as long as you find it relaxing.

So, breathe slowly and evenly, as in Relaxation Strategy 1. Then imagine you are somewhere calm and relaxing. Focus on this image, as best you can and in as much detail as possible. (Make it real—engage your senses and see, hear, smell, feel and taste elements of your scene. Be sure that you have put yourself in it.) Imagine everything around you is calm and relaxing. Stay with this image for as long as you can and, as with the other strategies, practice as often as possible.

## DISTRACTION TECHNIQUE

Apart from relaxation, another common strategy that can be useful is distraction. As with relaxation, the possibilities are endless. Distraction involves keeping your mind busy with something so long as it is not stressful or worrying. For example, thinking of something other than work or not sleeping is bound to be more helpful than lying in bed at night worrying about what you have to do and about being tired tomorrow (if this is a serious problem, Chapter 8 on controlling worry will be helpful).

The aim of distraction is similar to that of relaxation— to put stressful things out of your mind. With distraction, however, there is less emphasis on reducing tension and/or on feeling calm. Instead, the aim is to keep your mind occupied with something other than the worrying thoughts. There are many ways that this can be achieved and you may want to devise your own strategies. Here are some common methods that other people have found helpful.

The classic distraction strategy for sleeping is *counting*

*sheep*. Although most people think I am joking when I suggest this, it can actually be quite useful. The principle behind this is to focus on something monotonous and boring. Anything that is repetitive might work, so you could also imagine that you were walking down a long, straight road, with nothing but the white centre line to focus on. Or you could count the white posts that hold up the endless fence on the side of the road.

A similar approach involves using *number and letter games* to distract your mind from worrying and unhelpful thoughts. These can also be effectively distracting. One of the simpler and more popular ones involves working your way through the alphabet, one letter at a time, and thinking of animals or fruits (or anything, really) starting with each letter. For example, it could go something like "'A' is for aardvark, 'B' is for beetle, 'C' is for cheetah, 'D' is for dromedary . . ." You can continue this for as long as necessary. If you have completed the alphabet using animals, and are still awake, then you can start again, using fruits, or vegetables, or anything relatively unengaging.

Other strategies to consider include replaying a favorite movie in your mind or singing (not out loud, of course) a repetitive song. You could review the themes or content of a book you have recently read, or program you have watched. Alternatively, it can be helpful sometimes to shift your focus to something "outside"—staring at the ceiling in your bedroom or at some other plain and unstimulating surface might be worth a try. The options are endless. Remember that the main criterion is that you think of something to distract you from dwelling on the fact that you are not sleeping.

Finally, it is most important that you choose a relaxation technique that works for you and lowers your tension and stress levels. Once you start relaxing, you'll soon find that you're looking forward to your sessions and the improvements they make in your life.

# CHAPTER 6

# Sort out your sleep routine

## Sleep routine

Have you ever found yourself thinking, "there really must be a better way?" Have you ever thought "maybe I could do this differently?" Essentially we are creatures of habit. Even if we think we could be doing something better, more effectively, more efficiently, it is often hard to change old behaviors that have become entrenched and automatic.

Most of us, for example, like to eat our meals at roughly the same time each day and follow a regular pattern in the morning: when we rise, shower, eat breakfast and clean our teeth. The benefits of routine are plentiful. Regular routines allow us to perform many tasks and duties with minimal effort and with minimal thought. Regular routines can also minimize problems and maximize efficiency. Regular routines mean that you are less likely to forget to do something. When considering these benefits, however, we also need to examine whether the routine is really the most efficient and appropriate one for that particular task. It is good to occasionally review whether there might not be a better or easier way of doing things.

This applies as much to sleep as it does to other aspects of your life. Once you have a well-developed routine, you should find that sleep comes easily. Ideally, if you are sleeping well you should fall asleep within ten to twenty minutes of turning out the lights and lying down in bed. Further, all being well, you should sleep soundly until you wake in the morning feeling refreshed and ready for the new day.

Let's review and, where appropriate, modify your night-time routine and habits. It may be hard to teach an old dog new tricks, but it is not impossible.

---

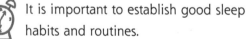 It is important to establish good sleep habits and routines.

- What do you do around bedtime?
- When do you go to bed?
- What do you do in bed?
- When do you get up?
- How long do you stay in bed?

# The sleep routine gone wrong

For a number of reasons, a poor sleep routine is a major contributor to insomnia. As mentioned earlier, sleep is simply not seen as a priority for some people and, therefore, does not receive adequate attention in their lives. In these days of globalization and 24-hour availability, work commitments have tended to blur into non-work time and night-time, meaning that for some people these have almost ceased to exist. The distinctions between work and leisure, work and home have become increasingly unclear in recent years. These and many other factors all contribute to the development of poor sleep patterns, which, in turn, contribute to poor sleep.

This may be the source of your sleep problem. Or perhaps a poor routine and bad habits have developed in response to poor sleep. In fact, you may have developed bad sleep habits in an attempt to cope with tiredness caused by a lack of sleep. Consider the following two examples.

> *Paul had recently been retrenched from his job and, although he was offered another position soon afterwards, there was a two-month gap between jobs. Initially, Paul enjoyed his enforced break, safe in the knowledge that he had something else to go to and that his redundancy package would tide him over until the new job started. He was for all intents and purposes on a paid holiday and he could see no reason why he should not enjoy it.*

*With nothing specific to get up for in the mornings, Paul began to sleep in and to rise later than normal. Because he had been working long and hard at his old job, Paul continued to go to bed at about the same time, catching up on sleep he had probably needed for quite some time. He thought of it as repaying his "sleep debt." In addition, because it was winter, he remained mostly housebound through the days, spending a lot of his time reading and watching television and videos.*

*After a few weeks, Paul found that he was not tired at his normal bedtime and he began to go to sleep later and later. Comfortable in the knowledge that he did not need to get up early for anything specific, he could see no problem with this newly developing pattern. At the same time that he was going to bed later and rising later, he began to take the occasional nap during the day.*

*After about a month, he found he was not sleeping at all well during the night and that he needed to compensate with regular daily sleeps. But this didn't seem to help and he found that he was not getting tired until very late in the evening. If he tried to go to bed at a normal time, he found he could not sleep and the more he tried to compensate, the worse his sleep became. Paul felt trapped and tired. As the start of his new job approached, he began to worry that he would not be able to manage at work. Not surprisingly, this worry did not help him to sleep either.*

*In contrast to Paul, Sonia's sleep pattern was not obviously irregular, but she found that her sleep was disturbed as a result of a very stressful period at work. Sonia had been working for several weeks on a very important project worth a lot of money to her company. During this time she had been working longer hours than normal, but more significantly, she had constantly felt under pressure and responsible for the project's success.*

*Not surprisingly, she found her sleep suffered, but this did not worry her significantly as she assumed that this was normal. She did begin to worry, however, when her sleep problems continued even after the project had been completed. She found that she continued to wake frequently through the night and that she was often tired during the day. The quality of her sleep was not as good as it should be or as good as it used to be. Accordingly, once her work hours returned to normal she tried going to bed earlier, hoping she would get more sleep. It did not work, and her sleep problems continued.*

*As Sonia's difficulties continued and as she tried to remedy the situation by going to bed earlier and earlier, she found that rather than improving her sleep she simply spent more time in bed feeling stressed and frustrated. She worried more about not sleeping and actually began to feel increasingly anxious as bedtime approached. As you might expect, this growing distress only further exacerbated her already troubled sleep.*

Paul and Sonia provide examples of two somewhat different ways in which a poor sleep routine can be associated with insomnia. In Paul's case, the development of a poor routine secondary to a change in his work (and therefore daytime activity and habits) led directly to difficulties with his sleeping. In Sonia's case, poor sleep associated with a common, normal stressor led to attempts to cope (i.e. going to bed earlier) that inadvertently disrupted her routine and contributed further to poor sleep.

 How's your sleep hygiene? (Do you have good sleep habits?)

Whether your routine caused your current sleep problems (as was Paul's case), or whether your routine changed subsequent to developing sleep problems (as was Sonia's case) does not, at this stage, really matter. What matters is that if you are not sleeping well, and if you have developed "bad sleep habits," then your routine is, at the very least, probably maintaining your sleep difficulties. What you need to do now is to identify where the problem lies and then do something about it. Developing good "sleep hygiene" (as the experts call it)—that is, good sleep habits—has proved to be one of the most effective tools we have available to help us get better sleep.

## Common problems

Before we examine what you can do to improve your sleep hygiene, it might be helpful to review and clarify the most frequently identified problems.

## IRREGULAR SLEEP TIMES

Sleep is, essentially, a behavior. As with other behaviors, it responds well to routine. Most people sleep much better when they observe a regular bedtime and settle into their own familiar bed. Disruptions to routine, caused by work, personal problems, or noisy neighbors, typically lead to disruptions to sleep. This does not mean you have to behave as though you are back in cadet camp, or under the thumb of a strict matron in hospital, or in prison—"Lights out!" There will be exceptions to any routine when, for example, there's a special night out, or you are traveling, or a member of your household is sick. Nonetheless you should strive to develop a routine and avoid going to bed at radically different times, as that is the way to wreck your sleep.

## IRREGULAR WAKING TIMES (AND SLEEPING IN)

Irregular waking times are probably more problematic than irregular sleeping times, because waking up later (sleeping in) tends to mean you won't be tired until later that night. If this gets out of hand, it can lead to a vicious circle developing in which you lie awake at night aware that you are not sleeping and so sleep in to try to catch up and reduce your sleep debt and your tiredness. Sleeping in, more often than not, simply leads to prolonged sleep disturbance.

## DAYTIME NAPPING

Similar to sleeping in, this is (in the majority of cases) just as unhelpful and ineffective. Daytime napping is perfectly understandable if you have not been sleeping well, especially if you are tired and frustrated. Sometimes all you want is a few minutes' sleep to recharge those batteries. But like sleeping in, although this might help you to feel slightly better in the short term, it almost certainly does not help in the longer term. The more you sleep during the day, the later it will be before you feel tired that night and the less sleep you will need that night. This just fuels a vicious circle and maintains sleep problems.

## TOO MUCH TIME IN BED

Even if you don't nap during the day, even if you don't sleep in, and even if you have an established bedtime, regularly going to bed too early can be just as troublesome. Spending more time in bed than you need to increases the chances that you will lie awake in bed worrying about not sleeping. This in turn can lead to your body and your mind developing an association between bed and worry. Clearly this is not helpful. Ideally, your bed and your bedroom should be associated with calmness, relaxation and falling asleep quickly. Scientific research suggests this may well be one of the most important factors at work in sleep problems (and therefore in treating and relieving those problems).

## TOO LITTLE TIME IN BED

At the other end of the spectrum is the problem of not spending enough time in bed, which obviously significantly reduces your chances of getting sufficient sleep. If you don't get enough sleep you will, quite simply, be tired most (if not all) of the time. It is important to ensure that you allow yourself the chance to get enough sleep and this will only occur if you spend a reasonable amount of time (preferably during the night) in bed.

## ENGAGING IN STIMULATING ACTIVITIES IN BED

As already noted, it is crucial that you develop an association between your bedroom and sleep (or at least relaxation). It is, therefore, important not to associate bed with any other activities, especially those that would be considered physically or mentally stimulating (the only exception here is sexual activity). With this in mind, it is generally recognized that among other things working in bed, reading in bed, talking on the phone or to your partner in bed, watching TV and/or eating in bed can all create sleep problems. Regularly having important (and potentially distressing) discussions with your partner in bed can be a problem. Certainly it is important that you communicate with each other and discuss matters of concern, but these conversations should not be conducted in bed nor, ideally, in the bedroom.

# Solution Part I – Sleep restriction

"Sleep restriction therapy" has been found to be one of the most effective components of treatment for insomnia. It is based on the assumption that in an attempt to cope with tiredness and to compensate for a lack of sleep, many people spend more time in bed than they actually require. They do this, not surprisingly, because they wish to sleep more, but this strategy frequently fails to accomplish its goal. In fact, in some cases the goal of sleeping more may actually be unrealistic. Scientific studies have found that many people with insomnia sleep more than they think they do and, in many cases, they sleep as much as people who don't report sleep problems. Many of these "insomniacs," however, take longer to get the same amount of sleep. What often happens in these cases is that spending more time in bed leads to a reduction in sleep efficiency. That is, more time in bed can lead to a poorer quality of sleep and, often, more frequent night-time wakings.

> Having trouble sleeping? Try restricting your sleep and spending less time in bed.

## THE AIM OF SLEEP RESTRICTION THERAPY

The aim of this therapy is to improve sleep efficiency and, consequently, to improve the quality of sleep. Initially, this may not necessarily increase the quantity of sleep, but as with lots of things, size isn't all that counts! And sometimes less is more. In fact, the initial phase of sleep restriction therapy requires you to reduce the time spent in bed, in order to ensure better quality sleep in the longer term.

Some people respond to the suggestion that they attempt sleep restriction with looks of disbelief, even horror: "How do you expect me to spend less time in bed when I'm telling you that I don't get enough sleep and that I can't cope as it is?" Many find it difficult to see the potential benefits of what is apparently a paradoxical, if not seemingly bizarre, solution—but it works.

## HOW CAN LESS TIME IN BED IMPROVE YOUR SLEEP?

The answer lies in weighing up the short-term versus the long-term consequences. In the short term, sleep restriction therapy may prove difficult and it may even reduce the amount of sleep you get, thereby exacerbating some of the problems you are having (such as tiredness, irritability and difficulty concentrating). But my clinical experience (supported by a substantial body of scientific research) indicates that these are short-term problems. In the longer term (which is usually within a few weeks), sleep restriction therapy frequently leads to significantly improved quality of sleep. In some cases, once the sleep restriction period has ended, there is also improved quantity of sleep.

Before beginning this part of the program, I often suggest to people that it might be helpful to think of other situations where they needed to take a step backwards before moving forwards. Can you think of a situation when marching directly forwards was not the best way to make progress?

Take this simple Rugby analogy. The best way to get to the goal line is not always a straight line forwards. If you are big and strong and fast this might work (a New Zealand All Black Rugby player of the mid to late 1990s, Jonah Lomu, comes to mind here). But not everyone can charge forward as successfully as Jonah did with his awesome natural talents. If you are smaller, there may be better strategies. For many, it might prove more successful to try to step and weave and, in some cases, to even go back and around.

Or consider a game of chess. Most of the more dangerous pieces on the board are able to move in any of several directions. One of the reasons that the king and the queen are valuable is because they can move forwards, backwards, sideways, and diagonally. These are potent qualities and are useful reminders of the limitations of simply charging on straight ahead (like the pawns).

## HOW DO YOU DO IT?

Well, once you've decided to give sleep restriction therapy a go, it is not actually that difficult. It involves working out a reasonable and specific amount of time to be in bed and sticking to that, regardless of how tired you might feel. The period spent in bed should as much as possible be taken up by sleeping, not lying awake in bed. Initially, it will probably be less time than you are currently spending in bed, but over the course of several weeks, once the quality of your sleep has improved, you can begin to increase the length of time you spend in bed.

To start with, you need to work out how much to restrict your sleep. To do this, you need to estimate how much you actually sleep on an average night. *Remember, this is the amount of time you actually sleep, not the period you spend in bed.* Any time you spend awake needs to be subtracted from the overall sleep calculation.

> Paul, for example, found in the early stages of his sleep problem that he would go to bed around 11 p.m. and rise about 7 a.m. This meant he was spending approximately eight hours in bed each night. However, Paul found that it took him about 45 minutes to fall asleep. In addition, he found that he was waking at least two to three times during the night, and he estimated that it then took about 20 minutes to get back to sleep. Taking this into account (45 minutes + 3 × 20 minutes =1 hour and 45 minutes), Paul was really only sleeping for about six and a quarter hours.
>
> In Paul's case, therefore, it was agreed that in the first instance he would restrict his sleep (and his time in bed) to six hours. It was then up to him to determine when this six hours (often referred to as the "window" of sleep) would occur. Paul decided that he would prefer not to go to sleep any later than midnight, which meant that he would then be required to rise at 6 a.m.
>
> Having decided on a midnight bedtime and a 6 a.m. wake-up time, Paul then agreed to stick to this plan for a week.

It is important to try this for at least a week because it can take a few days, if not longer, for your body to respond and adjust to the new regimen. Even if you are feeling more tired, it is important to do your best to persevere. Remember your commitment to the program and the reasons for beginning it. Think of the benefits you will experience when you do start to get better sleep. Remember that it is important to be realistic and that problems rarely improve overnight. With this in mind, it may be sensible to try this regimen during a relatively quiet week.

If you can stick to this for a week you should find that the quality of your sleep improves. You should also find that you wake less frequently and sleep more deeply, awaking in the morning feeling refreshed and energized.

Once this has been achieved, you can then try to increase the duration of your sleep. This should be done slowly and gradually and in a structured and routine manner. Typically, most people find that increasing their "sleep window" by about 30 minutes each week works best. Within a few weeks, you should find your optimum sleep time. For most people this will be somewhere between six and eight hours. You'll know when you've reached your optimum sleep time because you will start to find you are taking longer to get to sleep. When this happens, you might need to adjust your "sleep window" back a little (i.e. restrict your time in bed).

## TO REVIEW

Sleep restriction therapy involves a number of relatively simple, but structured steps:

1 Work out the number of hours to restrict your sleep to. (Note: It is generally recommended that you should not restrict your sleep to less than four or five hours.)

2 Set a specific time to go to bed and a specific time to rise, consistent with your sleep window.

3 Stick to this as much as you can, regardless of how tired you feel, for at least one week.

4 After approximately one week, and over the course of the next few weeks, gradually increase the amount of time you spend sleeping until you find your optimum sleep time.

## Solution Part II – Stimulus control

Along with sleep restriction therapy, another strategy directly aimed at modifying sleep routine is known as "stimulus control." It is also widely considered to be an essential component of any comprehensive sleep program. Whereas sleep restriction therapy attempts to tackle the problem of too much time in bed, stimulus control attempts to strengthen the association between bed and sleeping and eradicate behaviors that are not conducive to good sleep (such as worrying, working, reading or watching TV).

Stimulus control stems from what psychologists call "learning theory." That is, throughout our lives we learn to associate certain events and situations with specific responses. We don't always do this intentionally and may, in some situations, be unaware of the links and connections we make between certain things. For example, most people associate walking into a café or restaurant with eating. As a result, many people will begin to experience subtle physiological reactions consistent with eating as they enter a restaurant. As they peruse the menu, before they even begin to eat, many people will begin to salivate (some of you may recognize this example as being similar to Pavlov's classic experiment with dogs, which were found to salivate when a bell was rung because it was associated in their minds with feeding time). This illustrates the association we make between sitting in a restaurant reading a menu, and eating.

For a variety of reasons, people suffering from sleep problems have often developed unhelpful associations. That is, they learn to equate bed with worry or with stimulation from TV, books, and work-related matters rather than with relaxation and sleep. The ideal association between bed and good sleep has in many cases of insomnia been broken or damaged in some way. Instead of finding bed calming, people with chronic sleep problems often find it stressful. Instead of equating bed with rest, they associate (remember, not necessarily consciously) it with worry or with some other activity incompatible with sleep.

People who take work-related reading to bed, for example, may inadvertently come to link bed with work-related mental activity. For many people thinking about work is stressful. These people often wake in the night thinking about something they did, or something they need to do at the office. Similarly, without realizing it, many people who watch TV in bed can come to associate bed with stimulation. Many TV programs (and even the advertisements in some cases) are arousing and often contain emotionally distressing scenes and content. As such, watching TV in bed can lead to an association developing between bed and distress. Similarly, eating involves a degree of physiological activity and so those people who eat in bed are unwittingly conditioning their bodies to associate bed with physiological activity. Notably, none of these reactions—mental stimulation, emotional arousal or physiological activity—are compatible with relaxation or with good sleep.

The good news is that there is a way of breaking and of modifying these unhelpful associations. Some thirty years ago an American clinical researcher, Richard Bootzin, and his colleagues developed a set of guidelines that is still used today (with only a few modifications). Application of these guidelines has proved to be extremely effective for thousands, if not millions, of people with insomnia. Especially when combined with some of the other strategies described in *The Good Sleep Guide*, stimulus control can be a very powerful way of improving your sleep within a relatively short period of time.

Here are the rules, based on the original set of guidelines developed by Richard Bootzin and his colleagues. As well as the basic recommendations, I have provided a brief rationale for each guideline and comments on some of the more common problems raised by people who have tried to follow these rules.

1 **Go to bed only when you are tired and sleepy.**
This first rule overlaps somewhat with sleep
restriction therapy and is specifically aimed at those
people who go to bed early (either to sleep, read,
watch TV, etc.) hoping they will feel tired and fall
asleep. Usually, all this achieves is prolonged
periods in bed, particularly long periods in bed
lying awake and worrying about not sleeping. As
already discussed, this can also increase the chances
of bed becoming associated with wakefulness,
arousal and worry. Going to bed before you are
sleepy is simply not helpful. In fact, going to bed
before you are sleepy is distinctly unhelpful. Don't
go to bed if you are not sleepy; wait until you are
tired before retiring for the evening.

2 **Do not use your bed for anything apart from
sleep (the only exception to this rule is sexual
activity).** Do not read, eat, watch TV, or work in
bed. Ideally, don't do anything in bed except sleep.
Avoid your bed (and even your bedroom) during
times when you are not sleeping or sleepy.
Remember, the aim is to associate bed with sleep.
Conduct other activities elsewhere, preferably in
another room.

Remember that work-related activities or
anything that may be stressful or arousing should
not be engaged in close to your intended bedtime.
Ideally, you should leave at least half an hour to an

hour prior to your bedtime for winding down. That is, the last hour or so before you try to go to sleep should involve only relaxing, calming activities.

3  **If you find yourself unable to fall asleep, get out of bed.** Go to another room. Do something relaxing, calming, something that is not too stimulating. Do something boring. Do some ironing, read a magazine (not a thriller novel), look at a book that primarily has pictures. Remember again, it is important to avoid lying in bed awake and worrying. You should stay in bed only if you feel calm and relaxed. If you are in any way becoming stressed or agitated, get up. When you feel tired again (and only when you feel tired), go back to bed. If you are not asleep within 15 to 20 minutes, follow these recommendations again. Remember, the goal is to associate your bed with falling asleep relatively quickly.

4  **Repeat Rule 3 as often as needed.** There are, however, a few additional aspects to this strategy that you should keep in mind. Rule 3 advises you to get up again if you are not asleep within 15 to 20 minutes. While this is strongly recommended, it is also important to avoid falling into the trap of clock-watching (that is, the habit of checking the time every few minutes and thinking "I'm *still* not asleep"). Clearly this does not help, so beware.

There is an exception to this rule of getting up

and out of bed if you are lying awake: that is, if you are lying in bed, but feeling calm and relaxed. There may be no need to leave the bed if you are happily lying there thinking pleasant thoughts. In some cases, lying in bed in a relaxed state can be just as restorative as sleeping. If you are relaxed and calm, then fine, stay there. If you can use the strategies recommended in the previous chapter to help you to relax, then good. But if you find yourself worrying or becoming increasingly stressed and frustrated, then go back to Rule 3.

Note that following Rules 3 and 4 will affect your program if you are also attempting sleep restriction therapy. If, for example, you have set your "sleep window" at six hours and are following the rules above and getting out of bed when you are not having success at falling asleep, you obviously will not actually be in bed for the full six hours. This does not matter. Regardless of how many times you get up and out of bed, you should stick to your "window" of six hours. In other words, minutes spent out of bed are minutes when you simply miss out on sleep; the time at which you get up will remain the same.

5 **Get up at the same time every morning regardless of whether you have slept well or not.** Even if you are tired and feel you have not had enough sleep, it is important to stick to your

plan and to rise at the predetermined hour.
Sleeping in will only maintain your sleep problem.
Sleeping in is probably something you have tried
in the past and I think I am fairly safe in assuming
that it did not help or you wouldn't be reading this
book now. For most people it simply fuels the
vicious circle and stops them from feeling sleepy
at an appropriate time at night.

The idea is for your body to acquire a regular sleep
pattern. Normally this should come naturally, but if
something has led to the development of insomnia
we need, in the short term, to force the issue a bit. Do
not sleep in no matter how much (or how little) sleep
you feel you had during the night (the only exception
to this rule is if you have to do something, like drive
a vehicle long distances or handle difficult machinery,
that is potentially dangerous to you or others if you
are operating in a blur).

6   **Do not sleep or nap during the day.** The reasons
for this are essentially the same as those provided in
Rule 5. Some people can nap during the day and
still sleep well at night. For most people with sleep
problems, however, this is usually not the case and
daytime sleeping will negatively affect your night-
time sleep pattern. Similar to sleeping in, daytime
napping will disrupt your attempts to develop a
regular and healthy sleep pattern. Stay awake during
the day and, rather than sleeping or napping, try to

stay as active as possible (see Chapter 4 regarding the benefits of staying active and exercising).

## In summary

A healthy sleep routine involves avoiding excessive time in bed, and it involves using your bed only for sleep and sexual activity. If you follow the guidelines outlined in the two sections on sleep restriction and stimulus control, you will have a significantly greater chance of sleeping well and sleeping longer.

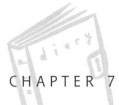

CHAPTER 7

# Organize
# your time

## Daytime connections to sleep

Many things in life are interconnected. It has been said that
there are only "six degrees of separation" between you and
anyone else in the world. That is, if you know someone,
who knows somebody, who knows someone else, and someone else and someone else, who knows someone else, the
last person in the chain of relationships could be the Queen
of England, the President of the USA, Mel Gibson, or anyone you care to name.

The point is that we are all connected, albeit distantly

in some cases. Similarly, it is true to say that all the different parts of our body are connected and interrelated in some way. The back bone is connected to the hip bone. Your eyes are "connected to" your brain which are connected to (or communicate with) the muscles in your fingers that are required to thread a length of cotton through the eye of a needle.

So, too, a range of factors can affect your sleep, and not just those that occur at night-time or just before you try to go to sleep. What you do in the morning could affect your attempts to sleep fifteen hours later. Your daytime is connected to your night-time. Almost all aspects of your life can influence your sleep.

 What you do during the day can affect your sleep at night.

The strategies and guidelines described in Chapter 6 are very important, but developing a good and healthy sleep routine depends on more than just attending to these areas. It also partly depends on developing a range of other behaviors (including organizing your daytime activities) that will be conducive to good quality sleep. If your day's routine is disorganized and hectic, your night-times probably will reflect this. If you have a stressful and unpleasant day, your night is unlikely to be much different. If you are unhappy and worried during the day, do you think you are going to be able to just "switch off" and relax during the night?

As we have seen in the previous chapter, people with sleep difficulties frequently develop bad habits at night. In addition, many of these people also engage in bad habits or problematic behaviors during the day. Often without realizing it, people with sleep problems are doing things and engaging in activities during the day that contribute to their problems sleeping at night.

We've already discussed how healthy sleep depends to a large extent on healthy living and how lifestyle factors, such as a balanced diet and a regular exercise routine, can help you to sleep much better. Let's now consider some common problems that tend to be associated with poor sleep.

The most common problem is attempting to do too much in too little time. Over-committing yourself can lead to work or other tasks and duties impinging on your relaxation and sleep time. Since this is such a common problem for so many people who suffer sleep problems, this chapter aims to help you to develop better time-management skills, as well as to provide you with ideas about how to get on top of other problems which may be disrupting your life and, therefore, your sleep.

## Time management

Learning how to manage your night-time and your sleep time will, in part, usually involve learning how to manage your daytime. A disorganized life without any routine is unlikely to help you to sleep well. At the very least, you should do all you can to ensure that your evenings are well organized and incorporate the proven and effective strategies described in Chapter 6. There is no doubt that a good sleep routine will lead to good sleep.

But achieving good sleep will often require more than organizing just your evenings. For most people, achieving a reasonable and organized routine during the day requires planning. For some this comes easily. For others (in my experience, the majority) who find it takes effort, thought and work, there are a number of relatively simple guidelines which, if followed, allow you to gain more control over your time and, therefore, over your sleep.

If you are constantly running late, pushing deadlines, rushing to complete assignments at the last minute, and generally feeling as though you are running flat out but not getting anywhere, then the following steps to achieving good time management should be helpful:

1 **Know what you have to do. List all of the tasks that you need to complete.** Depending on your situation, you might want to do this for the next day, the next week, the next month, or even the next year. How far in advance you do this for depends on whether you are having problems getting through your daily tasks, or whether your problem relates more to organizing things over a longer period of time.

2 **Prioritize. Ask yourself "Do these things have to**

**be done?**" Prioritizing is particularly important, because many people who find they "don't have enough time" frequently waste time on activities that are not essential or, in some cases, even important. If any of the activities on your list are not essential, then cross them off. But be careful—don't remove items just because they are unpleasant or boring. Avoiding difficult issues or problems will not make them go away. Only delete an item if it is genuinely not necessary.

3  **If you still have lots of things to do, consider your options.** If something does need to be done, do *you* need to be the one to do it? Could certain tasks be shared? Could some items be delegated to others? Could you get someone else to help you with some of the tasks or items on your list? At this stage it is crucially important to remember that there is only a limited amount of time in a day. There is a limit to what you can do and unless you are super-human, *you can't do everything!*

4  **Work out your timetable. When do these tasks need to be completed?** Now that you are left with only the important and essential tasks, take a clean piece of paper and write down the time by which each task needs to be completed. Does it need to be completed by 3 p.m., by Thursday, by next week, or not for three months? Try to be as accurate and realistic as possible.

5 **Work out your time budget. How long will these tasks take to complete?** Having completed Step 4, write down how long it will take to complete each task. Again, try to be as accurate as you can and to honestly estimate the time it will take you. It is a well-known fact that people who are often rushed or late consistently underestimate the time it takes to do things. If this describes you, make an effort to estimate the time more accurately and then, as a safety measure, add another ten to twenty per cent. It is better to overestimate the time it will take to complete a task. Then, if you have spare time left over, you can always do something else (or simply relax!).

6 **Decide when your plan will start.** Now you have a list of essential tasks, a time and/or day by which each task needs to be completed, and an estimate of how long each task will take to complete. Look at each task, one at a time, and work back from your deadline to determine when you need to start working on that particular job. For example, imagine that you have a project to complete at work, and you know that it will take you about three days to complete (factoring in that there will be interruptions, you will be required to do other things during that time, and given that you might need to wait for responses from other people— which, we all know, takes time). Let's say that this

job needs to be finished by Friday afternoon. Clearly you will need to have started the job by Wednesday morning (at the very latest). Similarly, if you have an hour of housework to do and you need to have it completed before your guests arrive at midday, you will need to ensure that you get started some time before 11 a.m. (again, this is the very latest you can leave it, since you might want to change your clothes and what if the phone or the doorbell were to ring and interrupt you!).

7 **Don't forget the big picture.** What you should have now is a list of activities and a list of starting times. Take each of these and list them in chronological order according to when you need to get started on each one. (Don't worry about the date by which they need to be completed.) At this point, you might feel the need to do some juggling. When you estimated the time it would take you to complete each task, did you take into account all the other tasks you had to do around that time as well? If you did not, then quickly review your list and ensure that you have allowed sufficient time for each task *given that you have other things to do during the same period.* If necessary, adjust the times when you should begin a task to allow for these other demands on your time. Again, don't forget that it is probably better to overestimate than to underestimate the time you are likely to require.

8 **Prioritize your priorities.** What if you find that you have more than one thing to start on a certain day or at a certain time? If this is your situation, you have several options. You can go back to Step 2 and consider whether or not both tasks really need to be done. Can one of them be shed? Or go back to Step 3 and see whether or not you could seek some help. Alternatively, you could prioritize the tasks. That is, ask yourself which one is really more important. If you can only do one of two tasks, you might need to make a choice. You can start with the more important task, or you can start with the one that will be finished more easily and perhaps more quickly. Sometimes it is easier to get started on something that is less demanding, and then move on to the more difficult task. Crucially, you will need to make a decision, and you will need to waste no time in getting started.

## Plan your day

Having worked out what activities you need to do, how much time it will take to complete them, and what tasks you need to start on certain days and at certain times, you are now ready to put together a plan. Planning your day increases the chances of actually achieving your goals. Planning your day realistically and specifically will increase your chances of success even further.

Planning your day involves *drawing up a timetable* with as much detail as possible. It is best to list as many things as you can think of and assign them an appropriate time slot. It is also important not to forget to include necessary breaks and other duties, such as having lunch and going to the bank. It is common to forget to include these types of activities, and to fill up all the available time slots with jobs that are deemed important and necessary. If you make this mistake, you run the risk of running out of time as you try to cram extra things into your timetable. So be realistic and don't fool yourself that you can do more than one thing at a time and still do it well and in a *calm, controlled, organized* fashion.

> "If you fail to plan, you are really planning to fail."
>
> —Anon

When planning your day and your week, it helps to include some *buffer zones*. These gaps or free spaces in your schedule will allow you to accommodate unexpected incidents or interruptions, and give you extra space and time in case an activity takes longer than you thought it would. You need these buffer zones to ensure you can cope with unpredictable events for which you hadn't budgeted. If you fill up every minute and every hour of every day, and then something goes wrong—a machine breaks down or someone is delayed (as often happens)—then you risk having all of your plans disrupted and being forced into spending the rest of your time rushing around trying to catch up. You guessed it, this is not good news for someone trying to achieve calm and control in their life.

If the term "catching up" sounds all too familiar, then plan to include several buffer zones to allow you the freedom and flexibility to cope with the many unscheduled and unforeseeable events that occur all too often. Remember, if you have spare time there is always something else for you to do. For example, why not use that spare time to practice your relaxation strategies, have a quiet cup of tea, or catch up on some reading?

# Just do it!

Did your mother or father ever stand over you, after having requested over an hour earlier that you take the rubbish out or wash the dishes, and demand that you "just do it now?" Despite the excuse that the task is boring or unpleasant, at the end of the day, nothing worthwhile is achieved unless you jump in there and just do it.

So having organized and prioritized your tasks, having planned your day and week, there is still one very important step. You need to put the plan into action, otherwise nothing gets done. Even with the most apparently overwhelming tasks, you have to start somewhere. Take one step at a time. Reassure yourself with the thought that every marathon starts with a first step. The key to success and happiness in life is often as simple as just getting on with the job at hand, seeing what needs to be done, and then simply doing it, no ifs and buts.

> If a task seems too daunting or overwhelming in its scope, break it up into smaller, manageable bits.

This applies to every aspect of life. A successful business does not simply happen on its own, it takes years of hard work to build it up to the stage where it is profitable. A satisfying relationship takes years of commitment and time and effort. A good level of fitness requires a devotion to regular exercise. Good psychological health demands constant attention and action from the individual. So do something—but ensure that you make the most of what you are doing by proceeding in an organized, efficient, manageable fashion. By getting your daily life organized, you are also planning for better sleep.

## Wind-down time

While we are on the subject of organizing time and planning your days, it is worth considering the types of activities that can induce good sleep, and where and when to do them. In general it is recommended that you have a "wind-down" period just prior to heading to bed to sleep. Consider the following example:

*When Sonia came to see me, I quickly realized that there was a problem with the way she organized her time. Sonia, however, could not see where the problem lay. When we discussed this issue she told me she was "very organized" and "very efficient." "Every minute of every day is accounted for," she informed me, stressing with pride, "I am so organized that I achieve twice as much as most people I know."*

*Yes, Sonia did organize her day efficiently and, consequently, she did achieve a lot. But time management, especially in the context of sleep problems, is not just about organizing every minute of every day. It is not just about maximizing your achievements. Time management, as far as we are concerned here, is about organizing your time so that you have enough time to do the things that will help you to sleep. A glance at Sonia's activity list will demonstrate what I mean. Consider Sonia's daily regime and see if you think it is conducive to good sleep:*

*Rising at about 6.30, Sonia would shower, eat breakfast and begin to prepare herself for the day ahead. During this time she would wake her three children and encourage them to get themselves ready for school. She would make their lunches and try to ensure that they did not miss the school bus.*

*Once her children were on their way to school, Sonia would head off to work, arriving at her office at about 8.30 a.m. On a typical day she would work through to 5 p.m. with only a half-hour lunch break. Because she had to leave promptly at 5 o'clock to pick up her children from after-school care, she was reluctant to take any more breaks during the day.*

She was determined to prove to her employers and colleagues that she could be as productive as they were—despite not being able to work back as late.

Once home, Sonia would help her children get started on their homework and supervise their after-school activities. During this time she would begin to prepare the evening meal. Although her husband usually washed up the dishes after dinner, Sonia was unable to take a break because there were still duties to complete—such as getting the children ready for bed and washing the clothes and ironing. Usually, the children would be in bed and the chores completed by about 9 p.m. For the next hour or two she would finish off work that she had not been able to complete during the day. By 10.30 p.m. or 11 p.m. she would be too tired to continue and would get ready for bed. When she turned off the lights at 11 p.m., she wondered why her mind was racing and why she found it difficult to sleep.

According to Sonia, her sleep problem could not be attributed to poor time management, because she felt herself to be very efficient and organized. And she did achieve a lot in the course of the day, in fact far more than most of us manage. She was an example of the classic "supermom." But she was also very tired, and struggling to maintain her exhausting schedule. How much longer would she be able to sustain this demanding routine? If she continued to be deprived of sleep, how long before something finally gave? Would it be her health? her marriage? her work performance? her patience with her children?

The problem as I saw it was not that Sonia was disorganized, far from it, but that she did not organize any time to wind down at the end of the day. As Sonia knew only too well, it is very difficult to just switch off after a long and demanding day of work—especially if that hard day extends well into the night. An active mind takes some time to slow down. There needs to be some sort of buffer zone between the stimulation and arousal of work and daily chores, and the state of relaxation and calmness usually associated with good sleep.

 30 to 60 minutes before going to bed, begin your wind-down activity.

A relatively simple solution involves planning an official wind-down period in which your mind and body slowly relax. This is your opportunity to let all thoughts of work and any of the day's stresses float away, and to allow more relaxing, bedtime thoughts to slowly come into your mind. Your wind-down activity should extend for at least the 30 to 60 minutes directly before turning out the lights and going to sleep.

Here are the sort of things you must avoid doing in your wind-down period:

- Avoid doing any work-related activity within an hour of sleep time.
- Avoid drinking anything stimulating (e.g. coffee, tea or any other caffeinated drink).
- Avoid vigorous exercise in this period before bedtime.

- Avoid engaging in mentally and emotionally arousing activities, such as reading thrillers or watching action-packed films or TV programs.
- Avoid any emotional or stressful discussions.

Here are the kind of things you can do to help you to wind down and relax:

- You could practice your relaxation technique.
- You could indulge in a hot bath.
- You could make yourself a hot, caffeine-free drink, such as warm milk or herbal tea.
- You could engage in a short session of gentle stretches to help release any muscular tension.
- You could listen to gentle music, but nothing too loud or upbeat.
- You could flick through a magazine, read or watch something on TV, so long as it is not too exciting or stimulating.
- You could even iron a shirt for the next day or engage in some mundane, soothing task (such as hanging up your clothes, straightening up a room, or washing your face and brushing your teeth). Basically anything that is undemanding, calming and conducive to good sleep.

 The wind-down routine is one of the most effective strategies for ensuring a good night's sleep.

At the end of the day, it is up to you to find what soothes and relaxes you. A calming pre-bedtime routine can easily be combined with the guidelines for sorting out your sleep routine described in Chapter 6. Developing and practicing a wind-down routine each night is one of the simpler strategies to be found in *The Good Sleep Guide*—and probably one of the more effective.

## Lack of pleasant activities

*Apart from having no wind-down period in which to let her daily and work stresses dissolve, Sonia suffered from another problem common to many people who have sleep problems. In fact I discovered a similar problem with Paul. Although not bearing the same parental burden as Sonia (Paul's wife was not working and so she was primarily responsible for what went on at home and with their children), Paul had more intense work-related stresses. As is all too common in professional circles these days, Paul worked up to sixty hours each week—and it was not unusual for him to take home work in the evenings and even on the weekends.*

*These hours were expected where Paul worked and it was considered almost odd if one was not seen in the office, at least for a brief period of time, over the weekend. Although well-remunerated for his efforts, Paul frequently felt that he had little time to actually enjoy the fruits of his labor. He had a nice house, his children had the latest computer games and sports equipment, and the family was accumulating a healthy bank balance, yet he often felt frustrated at not having the time to enjoy the benefits of his hard work. Essentially, there were very few enjoyable, relaxing and pleasant activities in his average week.*

*This was exactly Sonia's problem as well. Although both Paul and Sonia were achieving a lot and were successful within their chosen careers, they weren't actually all that happy. There were very few activities that either of them engaged in that were not related to work and duty. They had little time and energy just to be free to do whatever they chose. Also it is difficult to be happy if you can rarely relax for any sustained period of time. One day each week is not enough to wind down, especially if that day is a Sunday affected by the thought that "I have to go to work again tomorrow."*

At this point it is important to stress that I am not opposed to hard work, nor does hard work necessarily lead to poor sleep. However, I will repeat my strong belief, supported by sound scientific research, that good health—which includes good psychological health—is associated with good sleep. Poor psychological health, including unhappiness, depression and even boredom, tends to be associated with poor sleep.

Once again, the good news is that there is a relatively simple answer: as well as trying to ensure that you have a wind-down period at the end of each day, you should ensure that you are involved in some pleasant activity each and every day. This can significantly improve your mood and your general sense of well being. If you are feeling better, happier and more relaxed, you will almost certainly sleep better.

Moreover, it is not as hard as it might at first sound. Incorporating pleasant activities into your day does not have to require large amounts of time. Of course, if you have time available, then you only need to start determining to use it for your enjoyment—do as much as you can. If you have only limited time available, it is still possible to fit something pleasant into your schedule. One or two ten- to fifteen-minute sessions of pleasantness each day can make a substantial difference.

As with your wind-down activities, what you find enjoyable will depend on your nature and interests. It is all a matter of what works for you. If you are struggling to think of pleasant things that you can do in a short session, consider these possibilities:

- Take some time out from work and read the paper or a favorite magazine.
- Do some relaxation exercises, or go for a short walk and a change of scene and pace.
- Treat yourself to something you really like for lunch or your mid-morning or afternoon break.
- Leave your desk and have your coffee or tea at a local café.
- Arrange to meet a friend or co-worker (but make sure you don't talk about work or anything too stressful).
- Sit outside in the fresh air and soak up a few minutes of sunshine.

If you have more time, you could arrange on a regular basis to meet a friend for lunch or coffee. You can easily stimulate other interests and lift your eyes and thoughts from your work routine by visiting a local art gallery or museum. Why not join a club or adult education class that engages your interests in sport, history, music, literature, art, cooking or any hobby? If you look you're bound to find something to suit.

If you think these activities sound like a waste of time, consider the long-term and short-term benefits of feeling good. Consider what effect improved mood will have on your sleep. Once you are sleeping better, you will have increased energy and motivation to do more. It is paradoxical but probable, therefore, that taking time off to enjoy yourself regularly will actually reward you with more time and more energy. Once you start enjoying yourself, you will begin to relax more, and this can really help you to sleep better and, ultimately, have the reserves to achieve more.

# CHAPTER 8

# Develop healthy thinking and control worry

## Worry

As you've seen in the previous chapters, many factors influence our sleep. But the most common cause of chronic sleep problems is worry. The experts agree that worry (which includes stress, anxiety, mental activity that can't be switched off at night, and even depression) is a significant contributing factor for up to eighty per cent of people with insomnia.

Perhaps the most troublesome type of worry is that unstoppable mental activity that involves going over and over details (perhaps the past day's events or plans for the next day) when you are trying to sleep. Due to the pressures and stresses associated with busy lives which allow little time for relaxation, some people find that they simply cannot stop thinking (especially about any problems they are having) and that, consequently, they cannot sleep. These people often refer to their "racing thoughts." Not surprisingly, it is difficult to sleep if your mind is replaying or reviewing stressful events, or if you are mentally primed to anticipate impending problems all through the night. This kind of worry might initially disrupt sleep, but then the danger is that the sleep problem might be maintained or exacerbated by subsequent worry about not sleeping well. A vicious circle of worrying about worry or of fretting about not getting adequate sleep can develop, to the detriment of the poor, suffering, sleep-deprived individual.

> Worry (including stress and racing thoughts) is a major contributing factor to insomnia.

For most people, especially those suffering from chronic insomnia, worry is probably both causing and maintaining the problem to some degree. Most of the people I see who have been suffering from insomnia for many years report that in the first instance, a change in their life, or a specific stressor was responsible for disrupting their sleep. Despite the original problem having been resolved or no longer being relevant, they still frequently report worrying about not sleeping and, more to the point, worrying about the consequences of not sleeping. Either way, whether as a primary or secondary cause of sleep difficulties, worry does not help.

## Causes of worry

There are almost as many causes of worry as there are people with sleep problems in the world. Worry can be associated with almost anything. The more common worries tend to be associated with problems at work, problems with finances, or relationship difficulties. Slightly less common, but still prevalent, are worries related to poor health or illness, failure to achieve a goal, failure to find a goal, difficulties meeting deadlines or completing assignments/projects, and impending assessments or tests.

*Paul, for example, frequently worried about his work. All day and all night he worried about whether he had performed satisfactorily that day and whether he would perform adequately tomorrow. By necessity, his work required him to worry. Paul is a very successful broker in a large share-trading company and, to continue to be successful, he is required to be constantly vigilant to fluctuations in the market. Even a small change in the market affects whether and when to buy and sell. Missing an opportunity to trade can mean winning or losing many thousands (or in some cases many millions) of his clients' dollars. Being alert and vigilant (you could say, in a sense, worrying) are useful characteristics in his profession.*

As you can foresee, although these characteristics help Paul to succeed in his daily work, they do not help him at night. During the day when he is on the lookout for profit-making opportunities, his vigilance means he is less likely to miss out and more likely to catch the changes. But at night, with a mind that is still constantly alert and attentive, he often has trouble sleeping. As Paul knows all too well, it is very hard to relax and to get to sleep if your mind is in the habit of constantly reviewing the ups and downs of the economy and trying to predict future fluctuations.

Sonia is also a successful professional who, like Paul, works long hours in a job that most would agree is stressful. In contrast to Paul, however, Sonia is able to switch off when she leaves the office. When she gets home, Sonia is rarely plagued by thoughts of work. In fact, she usually feels relaxed and relieved on her way home and looks forward to the quiet hours in the evening when she does not have to deal with all the problems her job usually entails.

For many years now, however, she has experienced sleep problems. Although she does not worry about work, she does worry about not sleeping. As a result of not sleeping well for quite some time now, each night when she prepares to go to bed, Sonia begins to think about the night before and all the nights she has not slept well over the preceding weeks and months. She worries about not sleeping well and about what will happen if she does not sleep well. Sonia frequently worries that if she doesn't sleep well she will not be able to *cope the next day. She often worries that if she is tired, she will not be able to concentrate and to perform at work and that if this were to occur, especially if she failed to perform over a prolonged period of time, she would lose her job.*

Paul's worry about work and Sonia's worry about sleep were equally damaging to their night-time restfulness. As these two examples illustrate, it doesn't necessarily matter what you are worrying about. Whatever it is, worry will almost certainly disrupt your sleep. The problem to tackle is the primary one of the worry, rather than the secondary one of a lack of sleep. Worry does not solve problems and worry does not help you to sleep. In fact, if worry were an effective sleep remedy, then most insomniacs would never wake!

## Understanding worry

But not everyone worries. In fact, not even all people with sleep problems worry. Why then are some people prone to worry, while others appear relaxed and calm in the face of what appear to be similar stresses and strains? Why does Paul find himself worrying all night about stock prices and economic upturns, while other brokers go home and calmly sleep through the night. Why does Sonia worry when experience should indicate to her that worrying about not sleeping has not helped her?

There are a range of theories that attempt to explain why some people worry and why others don't:

- Some theories refer to genetic and/or hereditary factors, arguing that some people are simply born worriers.
- Other theories emphasize personality and suggest that different people are more prone to worrying than others. Similar in some ways to genetic theories, they suggest that each of us is born with a particular temperament and that essentially our personalities are determined from birth (or at least from a very young age).
- There are also theories that put our tendency to worry down to learning, and suggest that people who worry are more likely to come from families that worry. The assumption is that if your mother and/or your father were worriers, then you are more likely to learn to be a worrier.

There is evidence to support each of these theories. To some degree, contemporary research has found that worry can be attributed to genetic, personality, familial, and learning variables. Nevertheless, I don't intend to focus too much on all of these theories for one good reason: there is not much we can do about them. We cannot change our genes (not yet anyway!) or the families into which we were born and brought up. Nor can we, in the strict sense, change our personalities. But there is a very important aspect of worry that we can change: our thinking.

Regardless of the various contributions made by the aforementioned factors, it is interesting that not all members of a family worry. Even identical twins, with the same genetic make-up do not always experience equal levels of stress and anxiety. Individuals may find that they worry more or they worry less at different stages of their lives or in different situations. One of the most important factors that seems to differentiate between people who worry and those who do not, is thinking. Thinking, or your attitude, is a crucial determinant of the amount of distress different people experience at different times. There is always more than one way to think in any given situation and what we do know is that certain thoughts tend to produce more worry than other thoughts do.

> "tis nothing either good or bad except thinking makes it so'.
> —William Shakespeare, Hamlet

Despite the fact that we all live on the same planet and may even live in the same city, suburb, house, or even hold a similar job—some people are happier than others. Life can be an exciting and challenging adventure or a miserable, depressing drag, depending on how you look at it, that is, on your outlook or your thinking.

To illustrate this point and to see how this concept can specifically relate to sleep problems, consider the following:

*Paul and his wife Cynthia, who doesn't usually have trouble sleeping, both fall asleep. It takes Paul about 30 minutes or so, but he eventually drifts off following a busy and tiring day. He knows he will have another busy day tomorrow as there have been a number of important industry announcements that are likely to affect the markets and therefore his work in the coming days.*

*At 3 a.m. they both wake. Not surprisingly, Paul begins to worry about whether he will be able to get back to sleep and, if not, how he will cope the next day. He tries to relax, but finds he can't stop thinking about how tired he is, that it is only 3 a.m. and that he has to get up in three hours to get ready to go to work and then cope with the busy markets.*

*Cynthia also has a busy day tomorrow as she has a project that is due to be reviewed. She has finished most of it, but still has several hours of work to do to complete it and the review is at midday. Despite this and despite feeling slightly frustrated that she has woken at this hour of the morning, she lies back and thinks about her options. For a short while, she considers getting up to work on her project, but then rejects this idea because she predicts she would be too tired by the time of the review. Instead, she reassures herself that if she rises at 6 a.m. as she had planned, she will have enough time to complete the remaining work. In the meantime, she decides to enjoy the next few hours and determines to relax as much as she can. While Paul is worrying about having to get up in three hours, Cynthia is thinking positively about how nice it is that she has three more hours of rest.*

Check out your thinking. Is the glass half full or half empty? Are you a positive or a negative thinker?

Paul and Cynthia illustrate that almost every situation can be interpreted in a different way: it is the case of the half-empty versus the half-full glass. Although in this case the choice may seem trivial, in many others the choice is far more significant. In Paul's and Cynthia's situations, for example, the choice between focusing on "three hours of stress" versus "three hours of rest" could well make a substantial difference. While one may increase the chances of feeling tense and agitated, the other would be more likely to increase the chances of relaxation and thereby of sleeping. Obviously, the latter is far more likely to be conducive to good sleep.

What is important to note is that the way we think about things can make a big difference—to our overall happiness and, in this context, to our sleep. It is also important to emphasize that we can do something about the way we think about things. In contrast to genetics or temperament, which we cannot really change to any significant degree, we can learn to identify unhelpful thoughts and notably, we can learn to think in more helpful and less stressful ways. First, we need to understand why some thoughts are unhelpful and, once we have done so, we can then start to develop more healthy ways of thinking and of interpreting difficult situations.

## Understanding unhelpful thoughts

When I discuss unhelpful thoughts with my patients, they realize, more often than not, that these kinds of thoughts are indeed defeating. It did not take Paul long to realize that lying in bed thinking about how stressful his day at work was going to be was not constructive or sleep-inducing. So why do resourceful and intelligent people continue to think unhelpful thoughts when they are clearly self-defeating and damaging?

There are several reasons. One reason is that like many things you do, your thinking patterns tend to become habitual. Like a morning ritual of rising, dressing, eating breakfast, and cleaning your teeth, many things you do become automatic. If you do something often enough, it gets imprinted on your brain like software saved onto a computer harddrive. Once there, although it may be outside or beyond your immediate awareness, it can significantly influence your daily workings. In the same way, if you think something often enough, if you say something to yourself over and over again, it will continue as a thinking habit. Just as we develop and continue other problem behaviors, such as smoking, we can also develop bad thinking habits.

*Paul, for example, used to call himself "stupid" any time he missed a trading opportunity. On a bad day, he might call himself "stupid" ten to twenty times. To start with, Paul didn't really believe that he was lacking in IQ, but he did believe that it was imperative that he make the most of every opportunity and that to miss any would be terrible. Over time this tendency to call himself "stupid" became a habit and so daily, weekly, monthly, yearly Paul would berate himself. At the same time, he would do all he could to avoid being stupid, but that just made it all the worse when he did something that in his eyes was evidence of his ineptitude. Progressively, Paul felt increasingly inadequate and what were initially meaningless personally inflicted jibes, gradually became hurtful, self-defeating beliefs that chipped away at his confidence and self-esteem. The thoughts became more habitual, entrenched and automatic and therefore harder and harder to stop.*

> Are your thoughts your own worst enemy—undermining your confidence and self-esteem?

One of the reasons some people continue to think unhelpful thoughts is that they are simply not aware of them. The thoughts have become habitual, and many people rarely sit back and ask themselves "What am I thinking? What habits of thought have I formed?" In our society, considerable attention is given to emotions. Every day, people ask each other how they feel. Rarely, however, do we ask others in a personal context, let alone a business or professional situation, "What are you thinking?" or "What are your thoughts about this?" Many of the people I see for sleeping problems, when prompted to reflect on their mental habits comment, "I didn't realize I thought like that."

> *Before coming to see me, Sonia, for example, was not fully aware that she was spending so much time worrying about not sleeping and about the consequences of not sleeping.*
> *She was quite aware that she felt distressed lying awake at night and she was only too aware that her stomach churned and her head ached, particularly the night before an important meeting or an assignment was due. But prior to engaging in therapy, Sonia had never specifically reflected on the thoughts that raced through her mind while she was lying awake. She was, quite simply, unaware of how unhelpful her thinking was and of the negative consequences of worry with regards to relaxing and sleeping.*

However, there are other people who are fully aware of their thoughts and realize that their thinking is not helping them to sleep. These people tell me forthrightly that they know that they have negative thoughts and, furthermore, that they suspect that this way of thinking has a depressing effect on them. Unfortunately, these people believe that it is just the way they are. They feel helpless and incorrectly believe that they are powerless to change the way they are. Recent developments in psychological therapy offer considerable hope to those who want to stop worrying. There is a range of very effective strategies (mostly developed as part of the approach known as "Cognitive Therapy" or "Cognitive Behavior Therapy") that can help people to worry less and to gain control over those unpleasant "racing thoughts."

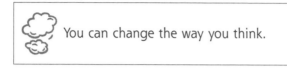

You can change the way you think.

## Common examples of unhelpful thoughts

Before we actually look at how you can change unhelpful thoughts and gain control over your worry, it is useful first to review some of the more common types of unhelpful thoughts. We are all prone to these, so you are certainly not alone. Though they are common, even relatively "normal," these unhelpful thoughts (which are often just misinterpretations of situations) can become intense and frequent, even habitual, and can have the power to subtly undermine your quality of life. That's when they become problematic. But it is important to remember that these bad habits can be changed.

How many of the following examples of the common types of unhelpful thoughts are familiar to you?

- **Catastrophizing** – This refers to the age-old problem of "making a mountain out of a molehill." Probably the most common type of unhelpful thinking, especially when anxiety and/or stress are involved, catastrophizing is the tendency to dwell on the worst possible outcome of a given situation. In addition to considering the possibility that something bad or unpleasant might happen, catastrophizing usually also involves the belief that "it will *definitely* happen and it will be *terrible*." Consider the following example.

*Sonia was lying awake one night worrying about the fact that she was not yet sleeping. In addition, she was also worrying about a number of things she had to do the next day. On this occasion, Sonia began to think about and dwell on what would happen if she were so tired that she was not able to complete these tasks. She imagined that she would be criticized by her boss and that she would be embarrassed in front of her work colleagues. Sonia's thoughts raced on to the point where within minutes she was imagining she would never sleep well again and, therefore, would not be able to function well at work. Consequently, she feared she would lose her job, be unable to meet her financial commitments and, ultimately, find herself destitute. Contemplating this sequence of events and this catastrophic outcome did not help Sonia to sleep that night.*

- **Selective abstraction and loss of perspective** –
  This involves focusing on one aspect of a situation while ignoring other (possibly more important and relevant) features. This is another very common form of unhelpful thinking, yet is one that often slips people's notice. Typically, when we are upset we tend to dwell on the negative aspects of a situation—ignoring or discounting other, more

positive, aspects. Along the way, it is easy to lose perspective and to perceive situations or difficulties as being far worse than they really are. Examples of how we select things out of our environment and range of experience are numerous.

Think of the last time you purchased, say, a new pair of walking shoes. Suddenly you notice scores of people wearing similar pairs down the street, in advertisements, on TV, whereas only the week before you'd been oblivious to them! Similarly, if you know someone close to you who is pregnant, don't you suddenly start noticing how many pregnant women appear out of the blue, and baby shops and strollers at the shopping centre? You may not be conscious of focusing on certain aspects of your environment that are of significance to you, but this phenomenon is nonetheless very powerful.

*Consider another example involving Paul, who has recently had a reasonable succession of restful nights. After a few good sleeps, however, Paul has a poor night following a stressful day at work. While lying awake, he thinks, "I'm sick of this, I never sleep well." Although it is understandable that Paul may feel frustrated in this situation, he is inadvertently engaging in selective abstraction or applying a mental filter. Without realizing it, he has filtered out and ignored the few good nights he recently had and focused exclusively on his current bad night and previous bad nights. Not surprisingly, this contributes to feelings of frustration and exasperation that are not conducive to restful sleep.*

- **Dichotomous ("all-or-nothing" or "black-and-white") thinking** – This is another pervasive and unhelpful way of thinking that we all engage in at times, although some fall into this trap more often than others do. Dichotomous thinking involves a person interpreting events in an extreme and rigid manner that admits of no middle ground. Anything that falls short of perfection, for example, is seen as a total failure. People are judged, often very quickly and on the basis of very little information, as either fantastic or terrible.

*For example, Paul engaged in black-and-white thinking when he said to himself "I never sleep well." Clearly this is an extreme statement, since he had just experienced several good nights. From Paul's perspective, however, he either always slept well or he never slept well. He was unable to see the "grey" and to acknowledge that, although his sleep was not as good as he would like it to be, there were times when he did sleep well. This example illustrates one of the common indicators of all-or-nothing thinking, the presence of "never." Dichotomous thoughts often include all-encompassing words such as "never," "always," "no one," or "everyone.".*

- **Setting unrealistic expectations** – This occurs when your goals are set too high, are too rigid and/or unattainable. Research suggests that people who do not become distressed often cope with problems by adjusting their expectations of themselves (and of others); they are flexible in their thinking. Worriers and those more prone to stress, anxiety and depression tend to set unattainable goals and are thereby destined to failure and disappointment. Unrealistic expectations are often reflected in inflexible thoughts that contain "I must . . ." or "I should . . ."

Paul, for example, had unrealistic expectations about how much sleep he needed. Many years ago he read in a magazine article that the average person slept for eight hours each night. After reading this, any night he slept less than eight hours he would worry that he had not had sufficient sleep. This would then typically lead to catastrophic thinking, during which he would imagine all the terrible things that would happen as a result of him not fulfilling his (expected) sleep requirements. (Note: In reality, although the average amount of sleep most people get is seven and a half hours, the range is considerable. That is, it is perfectly normal to sleep between six and eight hours. Some people simply need more, or less, sleep than others and there is no "perfect" number that applies to everyone.)

- **Overgeneralizing** – This occurs when you take a specific problem and interpret it as being indicative of a much more general problem. It also includes the tendency to "fortune tell," or to assume that because you have had particular problems in the past, you will continue to have these problems in the future. Generalizations can apply to people, to situations, to jobs, sport results—to almost anything. Overgeneralizing takes a single negative event and turns it into a never-ending pattern of problems.

*Paul's thought ("I never sleep well") reflects his dichotomous interpretation of past experiences. But then he went on to make an overgeneralization about his future prospects, moving from the fact that he was not sleeping well tonight to his extreme assertion, "I won't sleep tomorrow night, I'll never sleep well again." Sonia also illustrated this type of thinking when she got into bed at night and started thinking "Here we go again: another bad night, another tired day ahead."*

Before concluding this section, it is probably worthwhile reflecting on the fact that (as you may have noticed) most of these unhelpful thoughts overlap to some extent. Overgeneralizing and catastrophizing are similar. So too are catastrophizing and dichotomous thinking. It doesn't really matter all that much what you call these negative and extreme ways of thinking so long as you recognize them for what they are: unhelpful, distressing and potentially damaging to your sleep.

> Five names for unhelpful thinking:
> - catastrophizing
> - selective abstraction (loss of perspective)
> - dichotomous (black-and-white) thinking
> - unrealistic expectations
> - overgeneralizing.

## How to combat worry

If some of your thinking is unhelpful (which is the case for most of us), it will require dedication and perseverance to overcome this bad habit. Habits of thought, in many cases, have been present for months, if not years, so it is unlikely that you will be able to undo them overnight. However, it is important to assure yourself that you can change your thinking and that understanding and altering your thinking is likely to make a difference. There are three steps to helpful and healthy thinking:

- Learn to recognize the warning signs.
- Look for signs of the more common unhelpful thoughts.
- Learn to challenge unhelpful thoughts.

## 1    LEARN TO RECOGNIZE THE WARNING SIGNS.

Problems are easier to tackle if you catch them before they become entrenched. But recognising early warning signs is not so easy and straightforward. This is because many of our thoughts hardly surface into awareness as they race through our minds at lightning speed. Many thoughts are so trivial that we do not need to be aware of them. Even those that are more important can remain out of reach due to the fact that they have become habitual and automatic.

Even recognising the emotional warning signs can be difficult. Many of the people I see tell me that they don't realize they are getting upset until "it is too late." They report that they frequently only know they are upset when they are at the point of exploding. In reality, they don't reach that point of intense distress straightaway, but for various reasons, not being attuned to the build-up, they only notice the approaching crisis when things have become extreme and they have almost reached breaking point.

Consider a pot of boiling water. Slowly, the water particles accumulate heat and begin to move and, if you watch closely, you can see the heating water begin to swirl and tiny bubbles begin to emerge. Gradually, these bubbles increase in size and, notably, become more frequent. Eventually, large bubbles swirl rapidly. The water is now boiling.

If you compare stress to boiling water, then most people don't act to manage their stress until the water is well and truly boiling. If, however, your goal is to "cool down" before the boiling point is reached, then you will find it much easier to implement a plan for stress reduction as soon as you become aware of the stress equivalent of slow swirls in the water or those first small bubbles.

The first step towards healthy and helpful thinking, therefore, is to learn how to recognize the early warning signs that indicate we are heading down the wrong path. We all have different signs that indicate our stress equivalent of those small bubbles. We all need to learn to watch out for these and to learn how to recognize them early.

> Before we can change something
> we need to know what is going on.
> Develop an early warning system.

The earliest warning signs of stress and worry vary considerably from person to person. There are various ways of getting better at recognising these signs, but the most common strategies for increasing awareness usually involve becoming more aware of:

- your thoughts
- your emotions
- your physiological reactions.

The most obvious signs of stress usually involve some feeling of distress, accompanied by specific unhelpful thoughts and, at times, physiological changes (such as a churning in your stomach, sweating, an increased heart rate, breathlessness, and/or a "buzzing" or light feeling in your head).

One of the most effective ways of increasing your

awareness of these phenomena is to write them down. Keeping a diary has proven to be an extremely successful strategy for many people, helping them to better identify, and be alert to, changes in their thinking and their mood. You should try to make an entry into this diary as often as possible, at least once or twice each day. In particular, try to record any situations which cause you to feel stressed, anxious or depressed and, especially, any situations in which you are worrying about sleep (or about not sleeping).

To start with, divide a piece of paper into three columns. At the top of the first column write "Situation." This column is for you to record *where* you were and *what* you were doing when you felt anxious or stressed (e.g. lying in bed trying to get to sleep, or during an anxiety-provoking social encounter, or in a difficult situation at work). It may also be useful to write *who,* if anyone, you were with at the time.

At the top of the second column write "Feelings" (these are sometimes also referred to as "moods" or "emotions"). This column is where you record how you were feeling when you were in this particular situation (e.g. anxious, worried, depressed, frustrated, angry). You may, in fact, have been experiencing more than one emotion at the time. If so, record all the adjectives that apply.

Finally, at the top of the third column write "Thoughts." This is where you write down what was going through your mind when you felt anxious or stressed or what you were "saying to yourself." If you find this part of the diary difficult, ask yourself "What was going through my mind?"

By way of demonstration, one of the catastrophizing examples described above is shown recorded in diary form.

| SITUATION | FEELINGS | THOUGHTS |
|---|---|---|
| Lying in bed at night. | Worried and frustrated. | If I don't sleep tonight, I'll be exhausted tomorrow. I won't be able to function at work. My boss will be angry. |

In this example, it is clear why Sonia is upset and why she is feeling frustrated. On this occasion, she was concerned about what she perceived would be the probable negative consequences of not sleeping and of the impact it might have on her work performance.

In some other cases, however, it may not be as obvious why you are upset. Many patients tell me that they know they feel anxious, yet don't really know *what* they are worrying about. Sometimes they just "feel bad." At these times, if you are struggling to identify your thoughts, if you are finding it difficult to work out what you are really worrying about, try asking yourself these questions:

- What is it about this situation that concerns me?
- What's the worst thing that might happen?
  (The very worst thing!)
- What does this situation/event mean to me?
- What is it about this situation (or person or event) that I am finding so distressing?

If you are still finding it difficult to clarify your thoughts, then just try to write about the situation and keep writing. Sometimes, the real meaning of a problem comes out after you've been writing down your thoughts for a few minutes. Alternatively, try to talk the problem through with someone who knows you well and is close to you. Many people find that talking helps with certain problems, because when we talk things over we often clarify the issues in our own minds.

## 2   LOOK FOR SIGNS OF THE MORE COMMON UNHELPFUL THOUGHTS.

Having written down a few examples of situations, feelings and thoughts and, having become more aware of your feelings and thoughts, the next step is to take a close look at what is going on. In most cases, if you are feeling anxious or stressed, frustrated or depressed, you are probably engaging in one (or more) of the common types of unhelpful thoughts referred to above.

But remember, this does not mean there is anything wrong with you. It is common and normal to have unhelpful thoughts. Nevertheless, you don't have to put up with them. Take a minute to remind yourself that they are just "mistakes" and, like any other mistake, they can be corrected. Anyone can change their thinking if they understand how to do it and if they put enough effort into it.

Almost certainly it will take some determination to change your thinking. So now is a good opportunity to put some time aside to have a careful look at the types of thoughts that you have recorded. At the same time, refer back to the list of common unhelpful thoughts. Do you recognize any of these in your diary? Go through each of the thoughts you have recorded and next to (or underneath) your thought, write down the type of unhelpful thought (e.g. catastrophizing or black-and-white thinking). It might help to look for the following indications.

### Catastrophizing

This type of thinking is usually indicated by a focus on the worst possible outcome. Extreme adjectives and descriptors are often used when people catastrophise, so look for words such as "terrible," "intolerable," "unbearable," and "disaster." During the process of catastrophizing, it can be difficult to recognize the error of your ways, but it can be easier to look back on the thoughts some time later. An hour, or even a day, after the distress has subsided, review your thoughts and analyse them, paying particular attention to extremely negative words and phrases.

### Selective abstraction

Remember, this type of unhelpful thought involves a biased perspective. It involves looking at only one part of the picture. Selective abstraction is a form of losing perspective. Moreover, selective abstraction involves specific selection of negative aspects of a situation as opposed to the more positive or even neutral aspects. It is important not to blame yourself or to be overly critical. Rather, reassure yourself that this is not necessarily a conscious process. But do try to identify examples of selective abstraction, and of other unhelpful thoughts. To do so you might want to look for interpretations of events that seem to be too negatively and narrowly focused.

## Black-and-white thinking

As the name suggests, this type of thinking is usually fairly obvious and easy to identify. It might also help to think of the other names by which it is known: "all-or-nothing," "dichotomous," and "absolutist" thinking. Basically, these thoughts can be identified when words such as "all," "none," "always," "never," "everyone," "no one," "the whole thing," "nothing" are used. These thoughts tend to polarize at the extreme ends of a situation, and leave no room for any possibilities in between. They countenance no "grey," so to speak.

## Unrealistic expectations

These are usually reflected in the accompanying emotions. If you find that you are frequently disappointed and/or frustrated, it may be because your expectations of yourself and/or of other people are too high or unrealistic. It is important to recognize the difference between having high expectations and having realistic ones. Positive thinking and high expectations can be helpful, but only if you can actually achieve your goals. If they are realistic and achievable, then you are likely to feel happy and satisfied. If, however, you continually expect things that cannot be achieved, then you will suffer. These types of thoughts are often littered with words and phrases such as "should" and "must." These rigid and inflexible demands can be quite personally damaging.

### Overgeneralizing

This refers to the pattern of thinking whereby someone takes one example and concludes that whatever occurred in that instance has always occurred and will always occur. A single instance of a mistake becomes "all the time." One missed opportunity becomes "never." To identify this type of unhelpful thinking look for general, all-encompassing words in which a specific incident is taken to predict or sum up a much larger issue or problem.

So where are you now? You have learned to identify stressful situations and your feelings and thoughts at the time; you have also learned how to look out for some of the more common unhelpful thoughts. Although a good start, this is insufficient. You now need to do something about these unhelpful, unhealthy and self-defeating thoughts. You need to start to challenge thoughts that are contributing to your distress, adding to your worries and having a negative impact upon your sleep.

### 3   LEARN TO CHALLENGE UNHELPFUL THOUGHTS.

You can change your thinking. Even thoughts that have been around for a long time—long-term, chronic, and entrenched bad habits—can be modified. It is possible to change your thinking:

- if you know how and what to do
- if you are motivated and determined to do it
- if you persevere long enough to allow the strategies to be effective.

If you doubt your own ability to change your thinking, ask yourself the following question. Have you ever changed your mind about anything? Even if it was something that was not very important, even if it was only a minor issue, have you ever reconsidered something? Have you ever rethought your options? Have you ever recognized that you were mistaken and taken steps to correct that mistake? I'm sure the answer to all of these questions is "yes." Of course we have all changed our minds at some point in time, in some situations. In fact, if you think about it, we are constantly changing our minds. At times we change our minds several times a day, or an hour, or a minute! It may occur when deciding what you want to eat for lunch, or whether to leave work at 5 p.m. or stay back and finish off that project. How does it happen? How do we change our minds? If we can learn from these experiences, we should be able to apply the same, or similar, strategies to the process of changing unhelpful thoughts.

There are, in fact, many different ways that people change their minds. Sometimes, it just happens. A new idea pops into your head and you run with it. But more often it occurs as a consequence of deliberate consideration. You may consider a range of options and decide which is best for you at that particular time. It probably involves weighing up the pros and cons of each of these options, taking into account short-term and long-term consequences.

Sometimes, with the help of someone else, you might gain a different insight into the situation, or a new approach to or perspective on the problem. This may give you a more realistic approach than you are able to muster on your own —especially if the problem is personal.

Some people seem to be able to apply these thought-changing strategies naturally, while others need to learn how to do it or require the help of a friend to bounce their ideas off. Consider this example.

*Sonia frequently worried about not sleeping well: the more she worried, the harder she found it was to get to sleep. Consequently, she experienced increasing levels of tiredness and became, over time, irritable and stressed. In an attempt to cope, she tried to go to bed earlier—reasoning that she needed to catch up on the hours of sleep she thought she had lost—only to lie in bed awake for several hours at a stretch, worrying about not sleeping. Distressed at the thought of all the other things she could (and should) be doing with this time wasted in bed, Sonia's anxiety mounted.*

*When we talked through this situation, Sonia found she was able to modify both her thoughts associated with this problem and her approach to dealing with it. The first thing she was helped to realize was that her situation was not that* "terrible." We worked on putting her problem into perspective: although it was true that she was not getting the good quality sleep she desired, she was still sleeping enough to function, as her continued positive performance reviews at work indicated. Even though it was irritating, Sonia agreed that labelling her problem as "terrible" was not helpful and only contributed to her distress.

Once this was achieved, we began to look at how she was coping with her problem and whether it was working or not. Clearly it was not. We agreed, therefore, that a change was necessary and we decided that rather than just worrying about the problem, she needed to focus more on finding effective solutions. Her current solution (i.e. going to bed earlier) was obviously failing, so we generated a list of alternative options. In this case, discussion focused on the concept of sleep restriction therapy (see Chapter 6) and Sonia's problem was reformulated from that of not getting enough sleep to that of realizing that she was actually sleeping enough hours, but not efficiently. Subsequently, she agreed to try a different solution that involved actually going to bed later in an attempt to compact her sleep time and spend less time awake in bed. Going to bed later also allowed her to set a wind-down period during which she decided to engage only in pleasant and relaxing activities (which she had missed out on or had too little of previously).

Thus you can see how Sonia's more helpful attitude allowed her to use more effective problem-solving strategies to make a positive difference to her sleep. By putting her *problem in perspective, rather than catastrophizing, and by thinking about it in a different way and generating a range of possible solutions, rather than unhelpfully focusing on problems, Sonia was able to develop a plan that ultimately helped her. Sonia also benefited from specifically questioning and challenging her thoughts after being assisted to recognize that they were not helping her.*

You too can benefit from actively challenging your unhelpful thoughts. Here are some specific ways to challenge the common ones we have already discussed. To start, ask yourself questions that a kind and helpful friend might ask.

If you find that you are *catastrophizing* ask yourself:
- Is it really that bad?
- What is the worst thing that could happen?
- What are the real chances, or what is the probability, that this terrible outcome will occur?
- Is it likely, very likely or extremely unlikely? Has it ever happened before?
- Even if something negative could happen, does it help to dwell on it?
- Is there anything I can do to prevent it happening?

One of the keys here is to accept that your thoughts might be wrong. You might be mistaken, you might have misunderstood something, your thoughts might just be automatically or habitually unhelpful, or they may be distorted. Just because you think something, does not mean it is true or accurate. We all make mistakes and it is important that you are prepared to recognize these mistakes and to correct them. The potential benefits are enormous, so don't just accept every thought that goes through your mind. Question them, analyse them and, where appropriate or necessary, challenge them, revise or discard them.

If you find that you are engaging in *selective abstraction* ask yourself:

- Am I looking at the whole picture?
- Have I got everything in perspective?
- Is there another side to this?
- Could I look at this in a different way?

While asking these types of questions, some people find it helpful to imagine how someone with a different viewpoint would think if they were in this situation. If you know someone who seems to be able to keep calm and cope well with most situations, ask yourself how they would think about your problem. Could you think about it in this way?

The way to challenge *black-and-white thinking* is actually relatively easy: look for the grey. Ask yourself:

- Is there any middle ground? Is there a compromise?
- Is it really all or nothing?
- Is it possible that there are bits of black (bad or negative aspects) and bits of white (good or positive aspects)?
- Is it really that clear-cut?
- Could I be more flexible?

To start challenging *unrealistic expectations* ask yourself:

- Am I being realistic? Are my goals achievable?

- Is it helpful to aim towards something that may be unachievable?
- Would it be more helpful to break this goal down into smaller parts, into smaller, more achievable bits, into "stepping stones?"
- Do I really need what I think I need?
- Is it really so important that I, he or she does this or that?

You may prefer that things were a certain way, but are they really going to be that way? Remember that this world is not always fair and things don't always work out the way we want them to. Try to replace the "shoulds" and "musts" with "I would prefer . . ." or "I would like . . . but it's not the end of the world if I don't."

And finally, if you find that you are *overgeneralizing*, stop it! Instead, ask yourself:

- Does it help?
- If not, can I be more specific? Once you have specifically and clearly defined the problem, then do something about it.

But remember, one problem does not necessarily mean *everything* is a problem or vice versa. "One swallow does not a summer make," similarly, one problem does not a disaster make. One bad night does not mean you have never slept, or will never sleep well. So try to put things in perspective, be clear about what the problem really is and deal with each specific problem rather than overwhelming yourself with general worries.

In summary:

- Identify when you are stressed, upset or worrying.
- Recognize that distress is usually an indication that you need to do something and/or that you could benefit from changing the way you think about something.
- Begin to target problems and look for solutions.
- Identify what is going through your mind and write down your thoughts.
- Look for evidence of the more common unhelpful thoughts.
- Question them and try to think about things in a way that is realistic and helpful.

## Other thought-control strategies

In addition to the suggestions made above, there are other strategies that can help to reduce worry and to control unwanted, intrusive thoughts—especially at night when you are trying to go to sleep.

If you are continually worried about the time and find yourself frequently watching the clock, turn it around. Clock-watching does not help. Mostly, it only exacerbates worry, stress and frustration. If you are anxious about getting up at a certain time in the morning, set your alarm. The alarm will go off whether you are watching it or not (modern technology is wonderful that way!).

If you are concerned about how long it is taking you to

get to sleep, don't be, as it will take you longer to get to sleep if you are stressed. If you keep checking the clock, it will increase the likelihood of you having unhelpful thoughts such as, "Oh no, I've been lying here for fifteen minutes and I'm *still* not asleep." And how likely are you to get to sleep if you keep opening your eyes to peer through the darkness? Although it is hard, try to relax. Reassure yourself that relaxation is more likely to lead to sleep than is stress. Even if you don't sleep, relaxation is more rejuvenating than stress.

If you are worried about things you need to do the next day, spend some time before you go to bed planning and thinking about what needs to be done. Put into practice some of the time-management and problem-solving strategies covered in Chapter 7. You'll probably need to set aside at least a quarter to half an hour, and this should be well before the time you want to go to sleep. The idea is that you should deal with any problems before bed time. If you start thinking of things you have to do while you are lying in bed trying to go to sleep, remind yourself that you've noted it down and that you'll deal with it tomorrow, or later—*now* you are going to sleep.

So tell yourself that now is sleep time, not worry or work time. Remind yourself that if you get a good night's sleep, you'll be in a better position to deal with whatever the problem is. However, if you remember something important that slipped your mind earlier and you are worried about forgetting this idea or solution or feel it is going to haunt you and keep you awake, write yourself a note. Having done this, tell yourself that you will think about it and deal with it at a more appropriate time tomorrow.

> Useful tip: Keep a pad of paper and a pen beside your bed in case you need to jot down any last-minute reminders that might otherwise threaten to keep you awake.

As well as referring to Chapter 7 on problem solving and time management, it is also worth reviewing Chapter 5 on relaxation. There are times when it is best to simply focus on staying as relaxed as possible. It is not a good idea to dwell on longstanding or very important issues in the middle of the night. Rather, it's best to make a note to yourself to work on this problem later, and then to focus on relaxing for now.

At the same time, it is very important that at the first opportunity during your waking hours you do address longstanding issues, as they usually do not go away if you ignore them. Avoiding problems may seem to work in the short term, but in the longer term real problems will need real solutions and avoidance only makes things worse. Tackling longstanding problems may involve utilising some of the strategies described elsewhere in *The Good Sleep Guide*, or it may involve seeking professional help. Once again, there is no reason to think you need to solve all of your problems on your own. There are numerous services available (see

Chapter 9) and you should consider making the most of these services so as to fully benefit from this program.

Achieving good sleep is just as important as work and just as, if not more important, than many other areas in your life. In fact, it is good sleep that will provide you with the energy and motivation to be more productive at work and to cope better with your problems. Accordingly, time set aside for sleep should not be interrupted by other issues which are best considered or dealt with at other times. As mentioned, this may mean referring back to Chapter 7 to consider how you organize your days and weeks, and to assess how you manage your time.

Don't forget that it is important that you dedicate enough time to things that are important to you and that you devote sufficient attention and resources to improving your sleep.

# Deal with other problems

## The relationship between sleep and other problems

Poor sleep is frequently associated with other problems: in the daily routine; at work; at home; in relationships; or simply with sleep routines and bedtime habits. As we have seen elsewhere, good sleep typically depends on having other aspects of your life in order.

Sometimes sleep problems can be linked to psychological problems. This does not mean that if you are having trouble sleeping you are mad. What it means is sleep problems can be caused by, or can cause, emotional or psychological disorders.

For example, we all know that not sleeping well for prolonged periods can be frustrating and annoying. Moreover, it can be downright depressing.

Depression has a ripple effect which touches many aspects of your life, including your work and relationships. If your work performance or dealings with others are negatively affected, no doubt you will worry even more and become increasingly stressed. As stress builds, performance suffers and relationships become strained. Over time, each of these problems exacerbates the others, leading to a vicious circle in which good sleep becomes harder and harder to achieve as life's daily circumstances deteriorate.

Similarly, psychological problems can directly lead to sleep disturbance. One of the most common and significant symptoms of several psychological disorders is insomnia. For example, insomnia, is listed as a symptom of *major depressive disorder*. Difficulty sleeping also frequently accompanies *anxiety disorders, drug and alcohol problems* and is common in *post-traumatic stress disorder*.

Taken together, therefore, we can see how sleep problems can both cause and be caused by psychological disorders.

The good news is that there are effective treatments. All of the strategies outlined and recommended in *The Good Sleep Guide* will help you whether or not you have an accompanying psychological problem. If, however, you also

,

have other concerns, then it might be helpful to understand your problem(s) better and to be aware of the treatment options available. In "Further help and some tips" at the end of *The Good Sleep Guide* is a section for those thinking about seeking professional help.

# Depression

## WHAT IS IT?

Surely everyone knows what it feels like to be depressed. In fact almost everyone has felt depressed or "down" at some stage in their lives. But there is a marked difference between the mood or emotion we frequently refer to as "depression," and the formal psychological disorder that professional psychologists and psychiatrists refer to as "major depressive disorder."

The two are clearly related and most professionals subscribe to the view that major depressive disorder is an extreme, more intense version of the same, everyday problem of depressed mood that most people experience from time to time. But major depressive disorder differs in that it includes a range of other symptoms and associated problems beyond depressed mood. Depressed mood is obviously one of the core features of this disorder, but to be diagnosed as having major depressive disorder a person would also need to be experiencing at least five of the following nine symptoms, and these symptoms need to have been present for at least two weeks:

1 depressed mood most of the day, nearly every day
2 loss of interest or pleasure in all, or almost all, activities
3 significant weight loss when not dieting, or weight gain, or decrease in appetite most days
4 insomnia or hypersomnia (excessive sleepiness) most days
5 slowed responses or agitation or restlessness
6 fatigue or loss of energy
7 feelings of worthlessness and/or excessive guilt
8 diminished ability to concentrate or to make decisions
9 recurrent thoughts of death or of suicide.

Clearly major depressive disorder involves more than "feeling down." People who are suffering major depressive disorder also have difficulty enjoying things or gaining any pleasure from what would normally be pleasurable activities. They also frequently have trouble sleeping, often feel tired, and usually report having tremendous difficulties getting motivated. For people who are in the midst of major depressive disorder the smallest things seem to be insurmountable obstacles. Everything appears to be bleak—everything, including their lives, the world and, usually, the future.

And this is the key to understanding depression. Although many different theories have been proffered over the years, the one that has received the most scientific support is known as "the cognitive theory of emotional disorders." "Cognitive" refers to the way we think about things. It also includes our beliefs and the assumptions we make. It refers to the way we interpret different situations, as well as to the way we respond to and cope with the range of problems and stresses that we face from day to day.

> The way we think is central to our moods and our mental health. Negative thinking renders us vulnerable to depression. Positive thinking helps us to avoid depression, or helps us to quickly bounce out of a depression when it strikes, and prevents depression from becoming an entrenched state of mind.

In brief, cognitive theory proposes that people might become depressed for a variety of reasons, but that they stay depressed due to negative thinking. People who stay depressed for more than just a few days tend to be the people who place a negative interpretation on things around them. They tend to think that everything is bad and that they are in a hopeless situation. They are the ones who think that their coffee cup is half empty rather than half full. They focus on the problems in their life and find it difficult or impossible to recognize the good things.

They don't do this intentionally, of course, but they do it nonetheless and this habit, behavior or cast of mind significantly contributes to the extent to which they feel miserable.

Often, people who are depressed don't even know they are thinking so negatively, or, if they do, simply can't see any other way to think. Even if they are aware of the depressing nature of their thoughts and attitude, they find it very difficult to change, partly because they are so depressed.

What can also develop over time is a pattern of behavior that reinforces the person's beliefs that everything is hopeless and that life is dull and bleak. Many people with depression, for example, withdraw from social and recreational activities. They tend to stop doing, or do less of the activities that previously gave them pleasure. They avoid activities that in the past gave them a sense of satisfaction because "everything is so difficult and what's the point anyway?" As a result of this withdrawal and of the person's reduced involvement in pleasant and rewarding activities, their life really does become boring and depressing. It becomes a self-fulfilling prophecy. A person who believes that everything is miserable, doesn't do anything, and so their life does become miserable! The pattern of depression becomes reinforced and is maintained by both the negative thoughts and the self-defeating behavior.

## WHAT TREATMENTS ARE EFFECTIVE?

The good news is that there are a number of very effective treatments available for major depressive disorder. These generally fall into two broad categories: pharmacological therapy (medications) and psychosocial therapies.

The pharmacological interventions are most frequently

referred to as "antidepressants." These medications tend to work by increasing certain chemicals in the brain. In certain cases, this can lead to an improvement in mood within two to three weeks.

Although relatively effective in the short term, the problem with antidepressant medications is that they don't teach you anything about how to deal with or solve your problems. This might not be a problem if you are facing a stressful situation that will probably only trouble you in the short term and that will be gone once your mood improves. Unfortunately, many people who take antidepressants relapse once they stop taking the drug, because their problems remain unresolved.

> Antidepressants work while you are taking them, but cognitive behavior therapy teaches you how to cope all the time, with or without medication.

Psychosocial treatments, on the other hand, can actively help people with depression to learn how to solve their problems. The two most effective treatments—cognitive behavior therapy (CBT) and interpersonal therapy (IPT)—are aimed at teaching people skills, in a relatively short period of time, that will help them to manage better. Rather than directly solving a person's problems for them, CBT teaches people to act as their own therapist. Both these treatments are consistent with the proverb "You can give a man a fish and he will eat for a day, but if you teach him how to fish he will never go hungry/" CBT and IPT teach people how to fish, so to speak.

CBT and IPT are similar in that they both involve relatively short-term counselling (usually ten to fifteen sessions is all that is required). Both are structured around and focused on solving problems. They differ, however, in the specifics of their focus.

CBT tends to focus mostly on the nature of a person's thinking. It helps the sufferer to recognize the unhelpful, self-defeating pattern of their thinking, and then moves on to modify their thinking so as to develop more helpful, constructive thoughts. CBT also emphasizes the importance of recommencing enjoyable and pleasant activities. It encourages people to begin doing things again. This is not always easy when you are depressed, but it is possible—especially if the person is helped to take it one step at a time. Changing the way you think about things and changing what you do can significantly reduce depression and can lead to substantial improvements in quality of life (this is basically what we did in Chapter 8).

IPT, on the other hand, tends to focus mostly on the impact interpersonal relationships have on mood (and in particular, on depression). IPT is similar, in some ways, to the cognitive behavioral therapy for couples that is briefly described in the section on relationship difficulties on pages 197 to 203. There is a degree of overlap between CBT and IPT and the research seems to suggest that both are equally effective. Probably more important than worrying about which to choose is finding an appropriately qualified and experienced therapist in whom you have confidence and with whom you feel comfortable (see the section in the final chapter referring to "Where to get more help"). This person will be able to help you clarify the exact nature of your problem(s) and help you chose which treatment is most appropriate for you.

# Anxiety

### WHAT IS IT?

Like depression, anxiety is an emotion that we all experience to some extent. Like depression and major depressive disorder, feeling anxious is different to the formal diagnostic disorder of anxiety. To complicate matters there are at least eight distinct types of anxiety disorders recognized by psychologists and psychiatrists:

1 panic disorder
2 agoraphobia
3 specific phobias (such as the fear of heights or claustrophobia)
4 social phobia
5 obsessive-compulsive disorder
6 post-traumatic stress disorder
7 acute stress disorder
8 generalized anxiety disorder.

Because there is not enough space to describe each of these

disorders in detail, this section will focus mainly on those anxiety disorders that are more common and that tend most often to be associated with sleep problems. Nonetheless, it is important to acknowledge that any of the anxiety disorders, because they can be intensely distressing, can affect sleep. If you would like more information about any of these problems you should talk to your doctor and/or seek further, specialized assistance (see "Where to get more help" in the last chapter).

## PANIC DISORDER

The essential feature of panic disorder is the presence of recurrent and unexpected panic attacks. When these occur at night, they certainly can affect sleep. More commonly, however, these attacks occur during the day, but since they can have such a substantial impact on people's lives, they still have the power to significantly affect sleep. Panic attacks involve a discrete period of intense fear in which the person usually experiences intense physiological arousal in the form of an increased heart rate, palpitations, sweating, trembling or chest pain. These symptoms might be accompanied by dizziness, or feelings of unreality. Many people feel as though they can't breathe. Because they often don't understand what is happening to them and because the attacks strike without warning, people experiencing panic attacks frequently fear they are about to lose control, faint, go crazy, even die.

## POST-TRAUMATIC STRESS DISORDER (PTSD)

This occurs in a proportion of people following traumatic events. The most common example of a traumatic event is a serious motor vehicle accident, but PTSD can follow any experience in which the person felt threatened with serious physical injury, particularly if the event was perceived as life-threatening. Notably, not everyone who experiences a trauma develops PTSD, but those who do frequently experience heightened arousal and are prone to agitation, irritability and anger. They often report persistently re-experiencing the traumatic event in the form of nightmares and/or flashbacks. They suffer from repeated, intrusive and unpleasant thoughts about the incident that are difficult to ignore or control. Efforts to avoid reminders of the event typically fail and many sufferers of PTSD find that their lives become increasingly restricted as they try to escape triggering recollections.

## GENERALIZED ANXIETY DISORDER (GAD)

Sufferers experience excessive anxiety and worry about a range of events and/or activities. Whereas the fear in most other anxiety disorders is focused on a specific situation or event, people with GAD tend to worry about a lot of things. Moreover, the worry tends to be extremely difficult to control. GAD tends to be accompanied by restlessness and fatigue, irritability and difficulty concentrating. Notably, sleep disturbance is listed as one of the primary symptoms.

## WHAT TREATMENTS ARE EFFECTIVE?

Although the treatments for each of these three disorders (and in fact for all of the anxiety disorders) differ depending upon the specifics of the diagnosis and the individual variations that occur between different people, the scientific evidence strongly suggests that the most effective treatments are those generally referred to as "behavior therapy." "cognitive therapy," or "cognitive behavioral therapy (CBT)." There is little evidence to suggest that other forms of long-term psychotherapy or counselling are of any benefit.

As with psychosocial treatments for depression, the good news is that these treatments are extremely effective and achieve their results in a relatively short period of time (ten sessions on average). Although some medications help, CBT is just as effective in most cases and more effective for many people in the long term. CBT has very impressive long-term outcomes and significantly lower relapse rates than is found with medications.

As with depression, even when medications help people, they usually only work while the person continues to take the tablets. With CBT, however, the effects last beyond therapy because people are taught how to deal with anxiety (and with other problems) on their own. They learn active coping strategies that they can apply anywhere and any time (once they have practiced and mastered the strategies).

# Relationship difficulties

## WHAT ARE THEY?

Unfortunately, relationship difficulties do not really need to be defined because they are all too common. Surveys from a number of different countries suggest that relationship problems occur in thirty to fifty per cent of couples. Divorce rates in Western countries are soaring—and this only reflects problems between husbands and wives, not between non-married, co-habiting couples.

Relationship difficulties can also of course emerge between parents and children, students and teachers, siblings, employers and employees, co-workers, friends and neighbors, and so on. The reality is that people are prone to arguments on a regular, in some cases, daily basis. Some people do not get on well with others, and lack the basic skills to interact without friction and unpleasantness.

> Think about all the relationships you are a part of at home, at school, at work, in the neighborhood, and in your social circle. Do any of them keep you awake at night? Do any of them need improving? What can you do to make a positive change to your relationships?

Although theories abound and every relationship (however broadly defined) is different, there is an abundance of research suggesting that, at the core of many relationship problems, is an inability to communicate effectively. Aggression and passivity are unfortunately present more often than assertiveness. Yelling and screaming are more common than discussion and debate. Many people believe it is more important to achieve victory than to achieve compromise, agreement and a mutually acceptable situation.

Not surprisingly, if you are involved in a relationship marred by difficulties (whether it is with your spouse or partner, your parent or child, your roommate, neighbor, colleague or boss), then your sleep is likely to be affected. In particular, if a couple is arguing frequently, one or both partners are more likely to begin to experience depression. As already noted, depression is frequently accompanied by sleep disturbance. Marital disharmony (or relationship difficulties) and depression can also lead to changes in sleeping arrangements—the classic response of one partner "sleeping on the couch" is unlikely to be conducive to good sleep.

> When relationships are experiencing difficulties, sleep often suffers. Sleeping on the couch is rarely comfortable.
> In the doghouse, even less so.

Even if the disruption is not marital, but work-related or involving some other interpersonal relationship, the end result can still be sleep problems. This occurs because distress tends to be accompanied by ruminations about the source of the distress. If you are upset about Joe Blow, then you are more likely to think about Joe Blow. If you think about him, you remind yourself of, or revisit, your distress. A vicious circle gets under way, and as you become more and more distressed, you become less and less likely to sleep well. Interpersonal problems associated with work, business or social situations all have an effect on mood and sleep in a similar way.

## WHAT TREATMENTS ARE EFFECTIVE?

Finding the most appropriate and effective treatment will depend upon the exact nature of your relationship problem. No two couples and no two families are exactly the same. People's work and social situations vary considerably. Accordingly, there is no one treatment that will work in exactly the same way for all relationship problems.

> "All happy families resemble one another, each unhappy family is unhappy in its own way."
> —Leo Tolstoy, Anna Karenina

However, for most people in most situations the most effective intervention will be a psychological one that focuses on the way the various members of the relationship communicate and interact with each other. Consistent with the aforementioned treatments for depression and anxiety, the most effective therapies have come from the school of cognitive and behavioral interventions. That is, effective therapies for relationship difficulties tend to focus on what people do to each other and how each member of the relationship interprets and thinks about what the other has done. Consider the following example.

*Sonia began to develop problems with her husband as a consequence of being tired and irritable. Because she was not sleeping well, she tended to become upset more easily and over minor issues that would not have bothered her as much in the past. She tended to lose her temper more frequently and, especially when she was very tired, would argue more readily with her husband.*

*Sonia made repeated efforts to refrain from arguing, but found that she was just so tired that irritability crept up on her and got the better of her almost every time. She frequently apologized to her husband. Even though he was supportive and caring, and regularly told her that he understood how hard it must be not getting enough sleep, she often felt guilty and regretful afterwards.*

*As Sonia sank into depression, she began to withdraw from her husband thinking that this would be a way of avoiding more arguments. Sonia's husband tried to help by leaving her alone. He, too, thought that giving her time to cool off would be helpful for both of them and allow them to interact more calmly, even if less often.*

*Unfortunately, Sonia interpreted her husband's retreat as an indication that he was growing less fond of her, and that he did not love her any more. Sonia thought that the reason he was leaving her alone was because he was tired of her tantrums and she started to think that she might lose her husband—her only real support. Becoming more depressed, she also became more irritable. Her sleep deteriorated even further. Sonia began to spiral down into a deep, black hole.*

*Fortunately, Sonia and her husband sought help by going to a therapist who recognized that their problem involved a combination of sleep difficulty, mood disturbance and interpersonal difficulties. This was significant because, if they had seen a therapist who simply focused on the relationship issues, they might not have had much success. Sonia was unlikely to improve and be able to interact with her husband until she was feeling better and this depended, in large part, upon her sleeping more. As it was, Sonia and her husband received good help and eventually sorted out her, and their, problems.*

This example effectively illustrates how interactions between partners can become problematic. Let's briefly review Sonia's problem.

*Although the initial cause of Sonia's problems was her lack of sleep, Sonia and her husband's problems really started when she began to withdraw following the increase in their arguments. Although this strategy was understandable from one perspective, it was also open to misinterpretation by her husband. He thought that she wanted to be left alone and so did just that. From his point of view he was simply supporting what he thought was her decision to have some time out.*

*Although Sonia partially understood this response, she also believed that he was sending her an important message. She did indeed want some time out, but she also wanted him to keep loving her and to be there for her when she was ready to come out of hiding. When he wasn't there, she interpreted his absence as a sign that he had abandoned her.*

*The solution to Sonia and her husband's problem lay in exploring their responses to each other and their respective interpretations of these responses. This could only be achieved by communicating. Only then could they see which of the different interpretations was most helpful and accurate.*

*If Sonia's husband had asked her whether she wanted to be left alone or not, he could have avoided inadvertently upsetting her. Similarly, if Sonia had discussed her needs and talked to her husband about what she was trying to do and why she was trying to do it, she would not have unwittingly sent him the message that he should leave her alone. Neither spouse was right or wrong in what they did, but both made the error of not checking and communicating with their partner. They assumed without discussion that they were doing the right thing.*

 The key to stable and satisfying relationships is regular, frank, open and effective communication between the two parties in the relationship.

Avoid making assumptions and focus more on communicating effectively and checking regularly whether or not your partner is happy with the way the relationship is going. Good, effective communication tends to be the secret to good, healthy relationships.

And this does not apply just to marriages (de-facto or otherwise). It is relevant to almost any relationship, including the range of interactions that occur in the workplace. Although the nature of the responses and interpretations will obviously differ for work colleagues and employers, the basic concepts are remarkably similar. Interpersonal interactions tend to depend on interpretations of behaviors. The meaning we ascribe to what someone does is critical. It can mean the difference between a person angering you, simply irritating you, or not bothering you at all.

Solving problems in any type of relationship typically comes down to looking at what you are doing and at how you are reacting. It is also important to review how you think about and interpret the other person's behavior. Where possible, changing your responses and your thoughts can reduce the degree to which the relationship is problematic and can, therefore, reduce the extent to which you find it stressful. Ultimately, reducing your stress in these types of situations will help you to sleep better and that, after all, is your aim.

# Chronic pain and chronic health problems

## WHAT ARE THEY?

By "chronic" pain and "chronic" health problems I mean long-term problems which have persisted for more than several months and for which there is no cure, but which are not life-threatening. (Sadly, there are a number of issues to do with mortality and dying that make terminal illnesses and their associated pain different from what we are going to discuss, and that therefore require a different approach.) The most common types of chronic pain include lower back pain (which can follow a sporting incident, a fall, or a work-related injury), neck pain (which might occur following a motor vehicle accident), arthritis (which typically affects the joints and tends to have a gradual onset in later life), headache, and intractable problems such as asthma, diabetes and even tinnitus.

In more extreme cases, chronic pain can lead to a reduction in activity levels. This is not all that surprising because, if something hurts, it is understandable that the sufferer would wish to avoid making the movements that trigger the pain. The problem is, however, that inactivity can be self-defeating because with it comes physical deconditioning and, in some cases, depression. Both of these can then make it harder to engage in, or to enjoy previously pleasant and satisfying activities. Over time, a situation can develop in which the person's overall quality of life is significantly reduced and their level of suffering increases.

Whereas the mechanisms underlying many chronic pain problems are not well understood, science has made progress with problems such as asthma and diabetes. For the majority of people with these types of problems there are medications that can control the condition. However, for some these conditions can still be disabling and upsetting. Even conditions, such as tinnitus, that are generally considered to be not all that serious and certainly not life-threatening, can still be distressing. Sufferers tend to withdraw from social and recreational activities, not because it hurts, but because they have difficulty hearing and communicating effectively. As a result, they can become isolated and this leads to depression.

Although there are many people who live in hope, the reality is that at present there are no cures for many of these problems. The key point is that each of them can be managed and people can go on to live relatively normal and fruitful lives.

## WHAT TREATMENTS ARE EFFECTIVE?

In general, the same types of treatments that have been found to be effective for problems such as depression and anxiety are also effective in helping people to cope with chronic and intractable health problems. Cognitive behavioral therapy (CBT) has been effectively modified and adapted to help people with these conditions become as active and happy as possible, despite persistent pain.

Effective CBT focuses on helping people to develop

strategies to gain control over their lives. It focuses on teaching people strategies to manage chronic pain and helps them to develop a healthy lifestyle, including those aspects of diet, exercise and even medication use which will help them to cope best. Although CBT does not aim to cure, it can reduce the impact of these health problems on a person's lifestyle and mood.

There is a range of physical and psychological problems that can be caused by, or that can cause, sleep problems. For all of these, there are effective treatments. Some of the strategies described in *The Good Sleep Guide* can help, but if you are unsure how to begin managing your problem, or if you would like more information, consult the section in the final chapter, "Where to get more help."

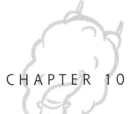

# CHAPTER 10

# Persevere and practice

## Perseverance

*Life is mostly froth and bubble,*
*Two things stand like stone,*
*Kindness in another's trouble,*
*Courage in your own.*

—Adam Lindsay Gordon

Morris Gleitzman quotes Adam Lindsay Gordon in his spoof self-help book, *Self Helpless*. Gleitzman remarks that "in the wee small hours, when I'm lying awake racked with worry and I've forgotten everything I've ever read in a self-help book, that simple verse often helps." How does it help? Well, by this stage you will recognize how the poet has captured at least two of the most important components of the Good Sleep Program.

First, in writing that "life is mostly froth and bubble" Gordon urges us to keep things in perspective. (Remember how in Chapter 8 we reviewed the harmful effects of catastrophizing? Things are often not as bad as we fear.) Additionally, the poet reminds us that it is important to help others and to be brave enough to endure your own troubles. And that's what this chapter is about. It is about sticking with the program through thick and thin. Many people start "lifestyle" programs, including weight loss and smoking cessation programs, but few actually finish. In these times of instant gratification, when many people hold expectations of immediate results (such as, speedy information-gathering on the Internet, or swift but complex calculations done with the help of computers), many find it hard to persist with things that do not work straightaway.

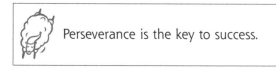

Perseverance is the key to success.

Expectations from science and from medicine are also very high. Almost every day we hear or read of fantastic breakthroughs and of new cures for complex and serious problems. Cardiac surgery is almost commonplace these days.

Organ transplants are incredibly effective and successful most of the time. People are being saved from what were once life-threatening illnesses, injuries and accidents. It is little wonder that people feel there should be a cure or "quick fix" for a relatively simple problem such as insomnia.

As with many things in life there is no miracle cure for chronic insomnia, it requires hard work, dedication and persistence. It demands the sort of effort required for achieving any other significant lifestyle change (such as losing weight, overcoming addictions to tobacco, alcohol, drugs, or achieving a greater level of fitness).

Not surprisingly, these types of programs only work if they are completed and maintained. Weight loss will not result from any program unless the participant adheres to the recommended diet and continues to exercise regularly. In the same way, the Good Sleep Program is unlikely to work if you do not continue to apply the strategies. Getting better sleep requires more than just trying these strategies. It requires maintaining the program set out in these pages for at least four to six weeks (in some cases it might not take this long, but in other cases it could require even more persistence). This chapter, therefore, is designed to help people to stick at it.

> If at first you don't succeed . . . try, try again.

If you cease to apply the strategies, then you risk losing the gains you have made up to that point, but by continuing to use them, then you should experience further gains and find the program becomes easier and more effective. As you persist and master the skills and strategies outlined, you should find that the program becomes a part of your normal life and, like brushing your teeth every day, you will be able to adhere to it without having to think about it much.

> About a month after agreeing to practice relaxation on a regular basis, Sonia found that she was relaxing without any conscious effort. Because she had made an effort to practice often, and to practice in a variety of situations and circumstances, she found that after a while it simply happened. As soon as she began to feel tense or stressed, she would slow her breathing, almost like a reflex action. As Sonia told me towards the end of her program, "I now do the relaxation without even realizing it—it seems to have become automatic."

This occurred directly as a result of regular practice and perseverance. All aspects of the Good Sleep Program can become easily integrated into your life—if you make the effort. With practice and perseverance you too can learn how to apply the strategies until they become automatic. Once this happens, you will find that your sleep improves dramatically.

## Practice

In the section on relaxation, the benefits of practice were emphasized. As noted then, relaxation is simply a skill, and, just like any other skill, the more you practice the better you will get. In the early stages, relaxation can be quite difficult for some people, but then so too can any other new skill or strategy that you are trying to master.

Think back to when you first started driving a manual car. Now try to remember how difficult it was when you first sat in the driver's seat and had to coordinate the various controls. As well as steering the wheel, there was the accelerator and brake to coordinate, not to mention the clutch and gearstick. In addition, you had to keep close track of the indicators, rear-vision mirrors and traffic lights. And you had to coordinate these tasks while listening to a parent or instructor provide you with advice and instructions every few seconds, while you manoeuvred a potentially dangerous machine down public thoroughfares!

It is not too hard to see that driving a car is an extremely difficult task. Yet, some time down the track most of us manage to drive with few, if any, difficulties. Over the weeks, months and years all of these seemingly separate tasks become easily coordinated until each is performed with little conscious thought. What were initially complex and overwhelming requirements have become easy, natural and automatic.

The process whereby the difficult and complex becomes easy and automatic applies to almost any action— whether it be driving a car, riding a bike, relaxing, mastering worry or developing a healthy sleep routine. Although some of the recommendations made in the earlier chapters might seem difficult initially, if you practice them regularly over a prolonged period of time, they too will become easy and automatic.

> Remember how difficult it was to balance a two-wheeler bike, or remain upright on rollerskates, or use a computer? Now think how much easier it became with practice.

You have mastered many skills over the years that are now second nature, but which at the outset were awkward, frustrating or difficult. Can you read? Write? Catch a ball? Tie your shoelaces? Walk?

Of course you can. But each of these skills was difficult in the first instance. How did you learn? Through practice and by making mistakes that helped you to learn and to improve your skills. Watch a toddler learning to walk and notice how often they fall over. And then what do they do? They get right up again and have another try. After a while, they are running around with a marvellous confidence.

By practicing and learning from their mistakes, babies learn how to walk. Expect to do the same thing when you start applying the strategies recommended in *The Good Sleep Guide*. You might stumble from time to time, but, if you get up and have another go, you will eventually master the skills necessary for good sleep. Stick at it and you will get there. Practice might not make perfect (remember that none of us sleeps perfectly every night of our lives), but it will certainly help you to sleep better.

## Make the program part of your life

If you think carefully about the other skills you have mastered over the course of your life, you will appreciate how easy it can be to master skills and then continue to apply those that are good for you. We tend to do this without always realizing it. Following a few simple suggestions makes it easy to incorporate a new skill and make it a regular part of your life.

Pause for a moment and ask yourself: "What do I do on a regular basis that is good for me and good for my health?"

I hope you have come up with at least a few answers, but if you are struggling, think of these relatively common and regular healthy habits: brushing your teeth to avoid the build up of plaque; engaging in any sort of exercise or activity; having an annual medical and dental check-up; eating fruit and vegetables on a daily basis; taking part in pleasant activities such as going for a walk on the beach. All of these are good for our health.

Do you perform these sorts of activities on a regular (that is, daily, weekly, monthly or yearly) basis? If so, how do you remember to do them?

Some of them you probably do without giving them much thought. Teeth-brushing has become so much a part of modern health care that it is easy to forget that it wasn't once so common. Due to massive public health campaigns, teeth-cleaning has become so routine that it is just a part of our daily lives. Most people do not spend time wondering when they will brush their teeth; yet we all do reach for the toothbrush in the course of the day. Generally, we get round to brushing our teeth because we have a set time when we habitually do it—it's probably been at pretty much the same time for years and years and years. It's a well-entrenched habit for almost everyone.

> Make your life easier and unclutter your mind of unnecessary thoughts: adopt a routine. Do yourself a favor, run through daily repetitive tasks on automatic pilot by instituting good habits that are set in a regular routine.

For some people, regular exercise and eating a healthy diet have become part of their normal lifestyle. They are not things they do when they feel like it, or when they get around to it. They are activities that are scheduled in, on a regular basis, to their daily and weekly plans. And because they have become routine, they get done more often. They are rarely, if ever, forgotten.

If you can apply this method to your sleep program, then you will significantly increase your chances of success. If you can coordinate and integrate your sleep program with your "life program," you will have a much better chance of doing the things that are required on a regular basis and you will give yourself the chance of mastering them more quickly. The sooner you master the skills and strategies, the more you will gain in a shorter period of time.

> Practice makes you better at what you do, and an established healthy routine allows you to practice more often with less thought and less effort.

So find a way to make relaxation part of your normal day. Set a time of day, or better still several times a day, in which you will practice your relaxation. Make sure these times fit in with your other activities and requirements and choose times when you are not likely to be disturbed. Ideally, set a time when it will not be impractical to relax. This means taking into account the normal, daily ebbs and flows of your home and/or your work life.

Similarly, set a time of the day and/or the week when you can exercise regularly. Remember that the goal is to be more active during each and every day, but also to engage in at least thirty minutes of focused and fairly vigorous exercise at least three to four times each week (essentially every other day). Finding the right time will again depend on your work and home commitments. It will differ from person to person. But if you can set aside a realistic time and stick to it on a regular basis, you will reap the benefits.

Most importantly, you should aim to develop an

evening routine that is conducive to good sleep. The main components of this healthy routine have been described in Chapter 6, but, as with all aspects of the Good Sleep Program, you will need to individualize it. You will need to take into account when you finish work; when you want to go to sleep; when your children, partner, roommates, or whatever, go to sleep; and what housework or other tasks need to be done in the evening.

> Your evening routine will need to consider the influence of any other people you live with, such as your spouse or partner, and take into account the time that they go to bed.

Although there are several factors to consider and accommodate, the benefits of a good night-time routine are enormous. Developing a healthy evening routine that is relaxing and calming and leads into restful slumber (as opposed to stimulation and frustration) can be one of the most important components of this program. Once you have developed a routine you believe will work for you, stick to it and try to ensure that you do all you can to make it habitual and automatic. Once you achieve this goal you will not want to vary it, except in exceptional circumstances, and you will find that like all habits, you will be able to stick to it without giving it too much thought or making a conscious effort.

# Use reminders

There are some things we do (such as visiting the dentist) which do not become part of an automatic, regular routine. We surely don't do it because we look forward to it and enjoy the procedure. So why do many people visit the dentist more or less annually? This is too infrequent to qualify as a routine and it is certainly not something that would be described as "practiced" or "skilled." Yet it is something that some people do regularly, without failure, and for good reason—they receive reminder notices in the mail or even reminder phone-calls. Every six months or so most dentists will call or send a message encouraging their clients to come in for a check-up. Now there are good health reasons for this, but this practice also makes marketing sense and is an effective way of reminding people to engage in a particular behavior.

What does this have to do with sleep? Well, you can use the same device—that of reminders—to ensure you engage in the behaviors recommended in the chapters you have been reading. You can remind yourself to practice the relaxation techniques, to exercise regularly, to work on stress management strategies, or to do any other things that you believe will help you to sleep better. You can also remind yourself *not* to do things if that is appropriate.

And the good thing is that you don't have to mail yourself a letter or email yourself a reminder! There are a number of simple, cheap and practical alternatives that you can begin to apply today. Follow these few straightforward steps and you will dramatically increase your chances of completing your chosen task and, therefore, of achieving your goals—which probably means you'll sleep better and feel better.

Having clarified exactly what it is that you want to remind yourself of, the next step is to summarize this task or activity in a few short, simple, positive words. A word or saying that is easy to repeat will work best. If, for example, you want to remind yourself to relax, then something like "keep calm" should work, or simply "relax" might serve best.

"Keep calm" or "don't panic" may sound like they are delivering the same message, but "Keep calm" is a better choice because the negative formulation mentions "panic" and the aim is to bring about its opposite—calm.

The next step is to decide when and where you are most likely to need this reminder. Trying to relax, for example, may not be necessary when you are showering first thing in the morning, but may be imperative at certain other times of the day in quite different situations. If your work involves talking to difficult people on the phone at regular intervals, then a reminder note ("Keep calm") just above (or even on) the phone would be helpful. If you tend to fall into a habit of worry as soon as you enter your office in the morning, then placing a note where you will see it straightaway (like on your computer screen or where you hang your jacket) would be a good idea.

> If you're shy about leaving positive affirmations ("Relax," "Keep calm," "Breathe deeply," and so forth) around your office or in sight of others, you could substitute bright, cheerful stickers, a "smiley" face, a picture of a flower or sun or something uplifting to remind you.

Quite simply, the idea is to place a short, simple reminder of whatever you want to do (e.g. relax or organize your thoughts) in a position where it will be most useful. It needs to be visible, accessible and easily understandable. It can be a few simple words on an adhesive note, or a more elaborate sign or notice that you design on your computer or using your calligraphy skills. It can be used at work, at home, in the car or anywhere. If you need something that is portable, you could place a small sticky dot (available at any drugstore or supermarket) on your watch or on your mobile phone, and use that as a reminder to relax or to leave work behind at the workplace.

## Schedule regular reviews

To review, you have begun:

- forming good habits that will become part of your daily routine

- using reminders to prompt you to practice your good behavior.

Another useful and important strategy to add to these is:

- reviewing your progress at regular intervals.

Almost everyone finds it hard to maintain lifestyle changes over long periods of time. Discipline is not the most natural of human characteristics. Even after months or years it can be easy to slip back into old habits. Only recently I was talking to a friend who had given up smoking for over three years when she started again! "Old habits die hard" and there are often frequent and powerful temptations to draw us back into our old, bad ways.

One of the other reasons that it can be difficult to maintain these types of programs is because any routine, even an effective and helpful one, can become boring and monotonous after a while. One of the riskiest periods for relapse is when you have achieved your goals. This is because having achieved your goals the motivation for continuing with the program has partially disappeared. It is, therefore, critical to continue finding new ways to motivate yourself and to continue redefining goals so you don't become vulnerable to old patterns of behavior.

One way of achieving this is to schedule regular reviews. This can be achieved in a number of ways, but most commonly and simply involves making an appointment in your diary for a time when you will assess your progress and review your goals. It will not work if you simply tell yourself that you will "see how things are going in a month or so." To be effective, you must actually write a specific time into your diary and stick to that time as though it were an appointment with an important medical practitioner or work associate.

> Make a date with yourself to assess your progress and brush up on any areas that need renewed attention. Write a time in your diary to sit down with The Good Sleep Guide for half an hour on a monthly basis. Once your sleep routines are well-established you may need to do this only every quarter or half year. But do ensure that you do it! So get out your diary and pen now!

Set aside at least half an hour (or more if you think you need it) and review your sleep program. The best way to do this is to skim through *The Good Sleep Guide* and briefly check how you are faring with each of the components. Pay particular attention to any chapters that you think have a special bearing on your situation and needs. Carefully review any sections that address any of the problems you are currently experiencing. If necessary, plan to spend time re-examining the relevant program components and/or restarting your practice of a particular skill or strategy.

In the early stages it is probably best to do this on a monthly basis. Regular, thorough check-ups will ensure you make and then maintain steady and continuous progress. As you get further along, however, you might consider reducing the frequency of your reviews and assess your progress every three to six months.

## Monitor for warning signs

It is most important when you are reviewing your progress to check that you are doing all of the things that are recommended to improve your sleep:

- Are you making sleep a priority?
- Are you eating a properly balanced diet?
- Are you exercising regularly?
- Are you practicing your relaxation techniques on a regular basis? Even if you think you have mastered this skill, it is important to keep practicing. If you don't, your skill level will drop and then you might find it difficult to apply if and when you need to.
- How are your evening and pre-sleep routines and habits? Are you avoiding any bad habits and have you replaced them with more helpful ones?
- Are you dealing with life's inevitable stresses on a regular basis? Don't let these problems and tensions build up. Tackle them regularly, while they are still small problems. It is much easier than allowing them to become bigger problems and having to deal with them then.

- Are you managing your time efficiently and effectively?
- Are you in control of your thoughts and are you thinking positively? Review the chapter on healthy and helpful thinking. If your thoughts are getting away from you again, then implement the strategies aimed at controlling worry. Question and challenge your thoughts and look for more helpful and realistic ways to think. Always ask yourself whether there might not be another way to interpret a situation and, if there is, whether there is a less stressful interpretation.
- How are you feeling? Are you functioning at your best at the moment? Conduct a brief psychological health check. Review Chapter 9 for common symptoms of depression and anxiety and check that you have not slipped into one of these conditions.
- Are you regularly practicing the Good Sleep Program strategies? If you are not applying a particular part of the program, you need to decide whether or not this part is important for improving your sleep. If it doesn't seem to be, then you may be able to pass over it. If, however, it is an important part of the program and you have drifted away from the healthy habits and routines that were helping you before, then this should be considered a warning sign that you are at risk of sliding back.

Regular reviews are opportunities to catch warning signs early (remember that bubbling water?). Intervening early will be easier than letting any of these problems develop. A warning sign could be:

- increasing caffeine intake
- taking work to bed with you
- sleeping in or napping during the day
- regularly eating a substantial meal a couple of hours before retiring for the night
- having racing thoughts or dwelling on incidents at night as you lie in bed
- drinking more alcohol at night
- growing levels of distress and/or worry
- physical symptoms such as a stiff neck, sore muscles, headaches, breathlessness
- irritability, moodiness, withdrawal, negative thoughts
- anything that suggests your mood and your sleep might be affected in a negative way.

Once you have identified one or more warning signs, it is important to act quickly. The sooner you get in and do something, the easier it will be. What you need to do will depend on the nature of the warning sign, but in most cases it will involve getting back on the program. This might be as simple as recommencing relaxation practice or it might mean going right back to the basics and reviewing why you should be making sleep a priority in your life. Re-reading *The Good Sleep Guide* at regular intervals, or at least dipping into the chapters that were most relevant and effective for you, is a good idea and will ensure that you don't forget any useful strategies.

## Elicit help from family and friends

A common mistake that we all make from time to time is thinking that we need to handle everything, every problem, on our own. Because we are afraid of appearing weak, needy or a failure, we often struggle on with our difficulties without consulting others or seeking help.

Yet there is so much help available that it is a shame not to use it at times. Especially that of family and friends. Often you will find that others have tackled similar difficulties to those you are facing and you can benefit from their experience. There is much to be gained and you will be conveying to the other person that you value their advice and are prepared to trust them with your problems.

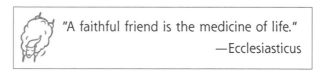 "A faithful friend is the medicine of life."
—Ecclesiasticus

Talking to someone about your problems can make the problem you are struggling with all the more manageable. This can occur for several reasons, one of which is simply getting it off your chest. Something definitely does happen when we talk about our problems. For one thing, when we put our problem into words, we gain a better perspective on the issues and a greater sense of control and focus. Afterwards things often don't appear to be quite as bad or muddled.

> Remember the wisdom of that old saying: "A problem shared is a problem halved."

So remember when working through the Good Sleep Program that family and friends can help by offering encouragement. Feeling as though you are being supported and being told that you are doing a good job can be very helpful and motivating. People close to you can encourage you to keep going through the difficult patches of the program when you might otherwise consider giving up. Family and friends can reassure you that your efforts are worthwhile, even when you are finding it difficult to see any gains. Support and encouragement can make an enormous difference when you are struggling to keep up a program such as this over a long period of time.

Having someone to talk to about your problems— whether it is sleep or some other difficulty—can also help if the other person offers you a different perspective from which you can view your problems. When you talk to someone else, they can suggest other ways of thinking about a problem or other ways of dealing with it that may be more effective and helpful and make the problem appear more manageable.

Finally, family and friends can help to remind you to

stick to the program and prompt you to do those components of the program that might prove to be helpful. Many parts of *The Good Sleep Guide* require constant attention and most of the strategies require persistence and practice. To master relaxation, for example, most people need to practice several times each day for several weeks. In order to develop a healthy sleep routine, to break the bad old habits and to develop the new good habits, most people need to stick at the program for several weeks. This entails remembering to do what's recommended and in the busy lives that many of us lead, remembering to do new things can be difficult.

One of the most difficult things to do is to change your thinking and, as was outlined in Chapter 8, healthy thinking is essential for healthy sleeping. This is especially true if you are, or have been, a worrier. Worriers tend not to sleep well, but worriers can learn to control the unpleasant and intrusive thoughts that so often interfere with their sleep. In order to implement the strategies that can help with this you need to remember what to do and be aware of when to do it. A close family member or a good friend can help. If they are aware of what you are trying to do, they can alert you if they think you are, for example, catastrophizing and becoming unnecessarily distressed. They can also remind you of ways to combat negative habits of thought, such as trying to keep things in perspective or considering whether the situation you are distressed about is really all that bad.

If possible, as a safeguard and to give you encouragement at crucial moments when your resolve may be about to waver, arrange for a family member or close friend to act as your Good Sleep Program monitor or reinforcer. This role involves keeping you on track when you begin to stray.

But in order for this to work well, your family and/or friends need to know about the program described in *The Good Sleep Guide*. They need to be made aware of the strategies that are effective. The more they know about the recommendations of the Good Sleep Program, and the more they understand your sleep problem, the more they will be able to assist. This means that you will have to discuss the program with at least one family member or close friend and explain to them what you are trying to achieve. Carefully choose your time to review the program. No doubt you will want to abbreviate the main points of it so as not to overwhelm them. You might consider lending them *The Good Sleep Guide* so that they can read it too.

Who knows, your Good Sleep Program helper or monitor may have sleep problems of their own, in which case you could help one another.

If you don't have a close friend or family member who can provide this type of support, then you might want to consider professional help. We all need help at times—there is nothing wrong with accepting it. If it is good help, it will be worth it in the end when you are sleeping and feeling better. Whichever approach you take, don't forget that you are not alone.

## Keep at it

In conclusion, it is important to keep at this program if you really want to reap the rewards. Giving up too early could mean that you never really know how good it could be. And it can be good. Good sleep can lead to you feeling better, having more energy and enjoying life in a way that you have only dreamed about! But in order to achieve these benefits you will need to be determined. You will need to do more than just read this book. For maximal gains, you will need to:

- read *The Good Sleep Guide*
- put the recommendations into practice
- and persevere for long enough (usually four to six weeks) for the program to become routine.

Once you have achieved this, you will be well on your way to a more enjoyable and fulfilling life.

# Further help and some tips

This chapter will consider where you can get more help and make some suggestions for sleep problems that occur in specific circumstances. These include:

- jet lag;
- sleep problems associated with shiftwork;
- sleep loss following the birth of a baby.

Essentially, each of these particular problems should respond to the Good Sleep Program approach, but there are a few tips and modifications to the basic program that are worth trying.

# Where to get more help

It has been noted that there are certain situations where *The Good Sleep Guide* might not be sufficient on its own:

- If you have seriously tried and persevered with everything in the program and are still distressed or not sleeping well, then you might need professional help.

- If you have any other significant health problems or are taking large doses of medication, then it would be advisable to seek professional assistance.

- If you think you might have any of the psychological disorders described in Chapter 9 (such as depression or one of the anxiety disorders), it is worth reminding yourself that there are effective treatments for these problems and that it is worth seeking specialized help.

Some people realize they need help, but do not know where to find it. One of the most common questions that I am asked is "Where can I find good help appropriate to my needs?" Unfortunately, there is no one simple answer to this difficult question. It is important to bear in mind that if you don't get what you want the first time, then try again. However, there are a few guidelines that should increase the chances of finding what you are after. Don't be afraid to talk to more than one doctor or psychologist in order to find a person and a service that suits you. Many different approaches are used, so be prepared to search around.

## DETERMINE WHAT YOU WANT OR NEED

The first thing you need to do is to think carefully about what you actually want and need. The answer to this question is often a more complex issue than many people realize.

For example, some people begin the Good Sleep Program so tired and frustrated that they have convinced themselves that anything is worth a try. Accordingly, they set off on *The Good Sleep Guide* adventure, determined to find the solution to their problems—only to discover that the solution is often not straightforward.

So when it comes to deciding what you want from treatment the first question is: Am I prepared to make some real and significant lifestyle changes? If you still want to, but have been unable to make it on your own, then keep reading. You might want to consider seeking the assistance of a clinical psychologist who is trained to help people make behavioral and cognitive (thinking) changes in order to achieve practical goals, such as sleeping better.

If, however, having read *The Good Sleep Guide,* you decide that this approach is really not for you, then you still have a number of options. The only problem is that you may have tried some of these already without success. Nevertheless, if you decide that what you really want is a "quick fix," such as a tablet that will help you to sleep more soundly and help you to get to sleep more quickly, then you need to talk to your doctor to review the available options and to weigh up their relative advantages and disadvantages. Be aware that the tablets that are available do not always work as well as people hope they will, or, if they do work well initially, tend to become less effective with time.

Your doctor will also be able to inform you of the appropriateness of a referral to a specialist sleep clinic. Most major teaching hospitals and some private hospitals have sleep clinics which are usually staffed by sleep specialists (often respiratory physicians) and sleep technicians. Sleep clinics will not be appropriate for all people with sleep problems, but could be significantly helpful for some in identifying, for example, such treatable problems as obstructive sleep apnea. Although this condition affects a relatively small proportion of all the people who experience sleep difficulties, it is a disorder that can be extremely disruptive and distressing and, notably, it is a disorder for which there is a relatively good treatment. An appointment and an assessment at a sleep clinic should be able to clarify this for you fairly quickly and so a referral should be considered, especially if you have tried many treatments without success.

## FINDING A QUALIFIED CLINICAL PSYCHOLOGIST

As noted above, if you are still experiencing sleep problems and are keen to resolve your insomnia, then I suggest you consider working through the Good Sleep Program (or at least certain components of *The Good Sleep Guide*) with the assistance of a qualified clinical psychologist.

*The Good Sleep Guide* is based on an approach known as "cognitive behavior therapy." Although other professionals practice this approach, *clinical psychologists* are among the best trained in the clinical techniques and, importantly, in the underlying theory. As such, a clinical psychologist will usually be the most appropriate person to help you with any of the problems you might be having putting the program into practice.

I have mostly referred to "clinical psychologists" as opposed to "psychologists." Both are licensed to practice—the difference is the level of clinical training they have received. Clinical psychologists have had at least two years of postgraduate training. As such, they are usually more skilled and knowledgeable in clinical theory and techniques. Therefore, try to find someone with a postgraduate degree, such as a Masters degree in clinical psychology (i.e. above and beyond an Honors degree).

Now where can you find a good clinical psychologist? Your doctor or general practitioner quite likely will have psychologists, physiotherapists and other specialists whom they can recommend or to whom they can refer you.

If your doctor does not have any clinical psychologists to recommend, then you will need to do some research of your own. One way to track down an appropriately qualified clinician is to call the national psychologist's organization (in Australia, this is the Australian Psychological Society). These organizations usually have a referral system that can guide you towards someone in your locality and/or someone with an interest in, and some experience in, helping people with sleep problems.

Alternatively, you could seek a more specialized referral by specifically trying to find a clinical psychologist expert in cognitive behavior therapy. Contacting the Australian Association for Cognitive and Behavior Therapy (AACBT) in your state or city should lead you to a CBT-trained clinical psychologist.

Another option is to contact a specialized sleep clinic and ask them for a recommendation. Although sleep clinics do not necessarily have a clinical psychologist attached to their team, they usually are happy to provide you with the names of clinical psychologists appropriately experienced and qualified in dealing with sleep problems.

Finally, if all else fails, you can always try the Yellow Pages telephone directory. This lists psychologists, although it is hard to tell which are going to be good for your needs. You can reduce the element of risk by choosing a practitioner from the section endorsed by the Australian Psychological Society (or similar recognized body). Although not an absolute guarantee of quality, it does ensure that the psychologist is registered and has at least the minimal qualifications necessary to practice.

> Where can I find a good clinical psychologist?
> - Ask your doctor.
> - Call the American Psychological Association.
> - Locate a cognitive or behavioral psychologist/therapist in the yellow pages or by searching the Internet.
> - Contact a specialized sleep clinic.

## DO YOU NEED OTHER SPECIALIST HELP?

Perhaps reading through *The Good Sleep Guide,* you have come to think that there are other related problems that might require some treatment. Let's say that your diet needs attention, or you are unfit, or experiencing bouts of depression or anxiety. Each of these might require a different treatment approach and a different clinician or therapist.

Depending on the nature of your problem, you might need to consider seeking the specialized help of a nutritionist, a dietitian, a personal trainer, a physiotherapist, a clinical psychologist, or a psychiatrist. As a general rule, a similar approach to that advocated above will probably help you to find your specialist.

So, start with your GP, who may be able to refer you to someone. Or indeed you may find the sort of practitioner you are seeking at your local medical practice, since, in recent years, many doctors have moved towards working in multidisciplinary group settings.

Or you could contact the governing body of the particular discipline, whether it is physiotherapy or nutrition, as most of these associations provide a referral service.

Where can I find specialist help?
- Ask your doctor.
- Contact the national body associated with your specialist's discipline.
- Consult with family and friends.
- Refer to the Yellow Pages.

Be prepared to search for a specialist who suits your personal needs and with whom you can establish a professional rapport. This may entail trying more than one qualified specialist.

Alternatively, talk to family and friends. There may be someone you know who has required the services of, say, a physiotherapist and who might, therefore, be able to make a personal recommendation.

However, none of these systems, even a referral by a national body such as the Australian Psychological Society, guarantees that you will like the person or feel confident that they can help you. And this is crucial to you overcoming your problem. It is essential that you feel relaxed with a professional and, most importantly that you respect their expertise in a particular area. Just because your doctor, your cousin or your co-worker recommends someone does not necessarily mean they will be right for you. If your clinician or therapist isn't right for you, then don't be afraid to try someone else. It might take a little longer, but it will be worth it when you find the right person and when that person helps you to overcome your problem.

## Dealing with jet lag

Travellers flying across time zones are all too familiar with the phenomenon referred to as "jet lag." It comes about due to the abrupt shift that occurs in your natural sleep-wake schedule relative to your in-built body clock. In simple terms, the enforced change that occurs in day-night cycles does not match the body's internal sleep-wake cycle and the body finds it hard to adjust quickly.

As a result of this discordance, many people experience exhaustion, lethargy and even some depression following long, transcontinental flights. Notably, however, despite feeling tired and exhausted, many people find it very difficult to re-establish their usual sleep patterns.

*Paul described this problem when he travelled overseas for business. He was required by his employers to fly to the USA for a meeting. He flew out of Sydney on a Monday and was due to attend a meeting in Los Angeles on Wednesday morning. He was then due to return to Australia on the Friday.*

*On arriving in L.A. Paul reported that he felt an "absolute wreck." Like many people, he found it difficult to get any more than fitful sleep on the plane. As such, he was tired and sleepy when he arrived in the USA, but he didn't want to go to sleep because it was early in the day. Instead, Paul reported that he made an effort to stay awake all day. He walked around the city and fought off the tiredness that was almost "overwhelming." Eventually, as night began to fall he relaxed and allowed himself to contemplate sleep after a nice dinner in his hotel restaurant. Over his meal he was so exhausted that he nearly fell into his dinner! Half an hour later however, much to his distress, as he turned out the lights he suddenly felt wide awake and no longer tired or sleepy. Paul found he was alert and energized. No matter how much he tried, he could not get to sleep.*

Although jet lag is simply a minor inconvenience for some people, it can be a major source of distress and disruption for others. In some cases, it can be associated with marked depression and even unpleasant physical symptoms (such as dry eyes, headaches, and nausea—although it is possible that these symptoms might be attributable to aircraft cabin conditions). In other cases, it can lead to significant impairment in functioning, meaning that the person cannot perform their job adequately (which is not very desirable for the person sent out to complete a project for their employers).

The severity of symptoms associated with jet lag can vary depending on a number of factors:

- your age (older people tend to be more likely to experience jet lag than younger people)
- the number of time zones crossed (as a general rule, the severity of the jet lag depends on how great the change in time is—in other words, how much the body needs to adjust its internal clock)
- the direction travelled (after travelling in a westerly direction, people are more likely to experience tiredness in the evenings and when trying to awaken in the early morning; in contrast, following eastward travel, people tend to experience difficulty getting to sleep as well as excessive tiredness in the mornings).

So, what can be done about it? Although there is no cure or sure-proof preventative measure for jet lag, there are steps you can take before you leave the ground and after you touchdown which will lessen the impact:

- **Do all you can to reduce your "sleep debt" prior to leaving.** That is, ensure you give yourself the chance to get sufficient good sleep before you go. You will want to follow as many of the suggestions in *The Good Sleep Guide* as you can for at least a week before you fly overseas. The better you sleep before you go, the better you will cope with the flight, and the quicker you will recover once you arrive.

- **Prepare for jet lag by anticipating time-zone changes before you leave.** This can be achieved by slowly adjusting your personal clock in the week preceding your travels. If, for example, you are preparing to fly to a time zone that is several hours ahead of yours, then you should, in the week or two preceding departure, gradually bring your bedtime forward (that is, make it earlier) a little each night and gradually rise a little earlier each morning. However, if you are flying to somewhere that is behind your present time zone, then you should try to go to bed later and rise later.

- **Similarly, you should try to function in your destination's time from the time of your flight or earlier, if possible.** If you can arrange it, one or two days before your departure you should adjust your watch to the time of your destination. From then on, you should try to sleep only during your destination's night-time and stay awake during your destination's daytime (regardless of the actual time where you presently are or whatever time it seems to be on the plane). To help with this, you can use eye-patches when you want it to be night-time.

- **Whether you sleep or nap during the flight will depend on whether or not you want or need to be awake when you arrive.** If you are going to try to go to sleep as soon as you arrive at your destination, then you might want to try staying awake as much as you can in order to facilitate going to sleep on arrival—unless, of course, you are on a 15-hour-plus flight, in which case you should try to get some sleep at the very least. Alternatively, if you need to be awake and alert when you arrive you should try to sleep as much as possible during the flight.

- **Try to organize business appointments or other commitments for times when you are most likely to be awake and functioning.** This involves trying to predict when you are likely to be alert in your destination. If, for example, you are likely to need to go to sleep later and rise later than you do normally, then try to avoid scheduling early-morning meetings.

- **Try to avoid caffeine and alcohol during the period of time you are flying.** It is generally suggested that you should avoid alcohol while flying as it can be dehydrating. Similarly, it is often recommended that you *avoid heavy meals*, and only eat light snacks while travelling over long distances. Instead, try to *drink lots of water*, and stick to plain (rather than exotic) foods.

- **Do your best to make yourself comfortable during a long flight.** Airline seats are not known for being conducive to good sleeping, and so you may want to make some modifications. Placing a small pillow (or a jumper or airline blanket) behind your lower back can provide much-needed support. Similarly, a neck pillow or one of those U-shaped inflatable pillows can be very helpful.

- Get up at regular intervals and move about the plane to help your circulation.

An important factor that is often ignored is how long you are staying at your destination. Although the recommendations above encourage you to adjust to your destination's time zone, this might not always be the best option. If you are staying somewhere for a reasonably long period of time then, certainly, adjusting your time clock will be necessary. If, however, you are making a short business trip of only a few days, it might be worth sticking to your home time and trying to organize yourself as much as possible within your normal time frame (e.g. try to only organize late-afternoon appointments if this is when you are more likely to be awake and alert).

## Coping with shiftwork

The effects of shiftwork are very similar to those of jet lag. Not surprisingly, therefore, the strategies that help with jet lag can also help with shiftwork. Shiftwork can affect sleep in several ways. The most common effect is due to changing patterns. Shiftworkers often do not work the same timetable on a regular basis. Rather, they might work early mornings one week and then late nights the next week. This makes it very difficult (if not impossible) to develop a routine.

At the same time, shiftwork can cause problems when it

robs people of their exposure to normal daily fluctuations in temperature and, more importantly, light. Often, shiftworkers working at night will try to sleep during the day which, although understandable, means that they are not exposed to natural light. This can be important since natural light and changes in light are part of what sets our body clocks which influences the flow and release of certain chemicals in the body.

Whatever the cause, shiftwork can frequently be associated with tiredness, which, in turn, can be associated with impaired performance. This can be particularly dangerous if workers are involved in operating machinery and/or if they are required to drive to or from work. In either situation, tiredness can increase the chances of accidents, which can then contribute to work-related or motor-vehicle accidents.

Theoretically, workers could adjust to shiftwork schedules if they simply adapted their lifestyles to, say, working at night and sleeping during the day. And this is exactly what many try, with some success. The problem comes about, however, because very few workers are able to completely adjust their lifestyles and fewer still are able to maintain this alternative cycle for prolonged periods.

Instead, what tends to happen is that employers change workers' schedules every week or so—just when they have begun to get used to the timetable. Further, many workers break their routine on weekends (or off-days) so that they can see family and friends during more standard hours. As a result, they never really stick to a routine for long enough. Rather shiftworkers chop and change between different routines.

> Follow the clock!
> Research shows that it is easier to cope with forward (or clockwise) changes in schedule as opposed to backwards (or anti-clockwise) changes. So, rather than changing from an evening to an afternoon shift, it would be recommended that shifts change from, say, afternoon to evening, evening to night, or night to day shifts. Employers should note that these types of changes can lead to lower rates of absenteeism and increases in productivity.

Despite these difficulties, there are ways of coping with shiftwork, although it needs to be noted that many workers do not have complete control over their own lifestyles. It is hoped that some employers and managers might read this, take heed of the suggestions, and make changes that, in parts of the world, have been adapted with great success.

The first thing that the worker can do is to try to follow as much of *The Good Sleep Guide* as possible, whenever possible. That is, even if you can't adhere to all of the recommendations in this guide, something is usually better than nothing. Try to practice as much as you can. Strategies such as relaxation, regular exercise, diet and stress management are all useful, regardless of the hours you work. At the same time, the sleep routine suggestions can obviously be harder to manage.

Despite this, try to do the best you can as often as you can to develop a healthy and regular sleep pattern. If your work schedule changes frequently, you could also try some of the suggestions noted above that are aimed at dealing with jet lag. Adjusting to different time zones is not dissimilar to adjusting to different work timetables.

In addition to trying these suggestions, you could try talking to your boss or your manager to see if they are willing to consider the good evidence that suggests that shift changes every three to four weeks is much easier on workers than more frequent changes. This allows workers longer to adjust to and settle into the new timetable, as well as meaning that they need to adjust less often. And fewer adjustments mean less tiredness, fewer chances of accidents and mistakes, and a happier, healthier staff.

## Following the birth of a baby

There is one last situation that is frequently associated with disturbed sleep. Although many people with sleep problems state that they would love to "sleep like a baby," anyone who has had one knows that newborn babies sleep for only short periods of time, waking often for feeding. What this means is that new mothers (and sometimes fathers) are frequently woken, often every few hours, to care for their dependent child.

Although most new parents are more than happy and willing to perform the necessary duties and to care for their child, the impact this has on their sleep can be extremely difficult to cope with at times. Sleep loss is significant in some cases and, it is not surprising, therefore, that some parents experience marked mood disturbance, find it difficult to manage, are irritable, or even depressed.

Most parents will get along without any real need of extra help or guidance. However, there are some strategies that can make it easier for new parents, allowing them a better chance to enjoy their babies and their early years together.

The relevance of the following strategies, however, will depend partly on whether you decide to breastfeed your child or not. Without getting into a discussion on the pros and cons of breastfeeding, this is an important decision to make from the point of view of sleep, as it will determine how much of the caring can be shared by the parents. Clearly, if you choose to breastfeed, then the extent to which the father can help becomes limited. Some couples institute a system whereby the father changes the diapers at night and carries the baby to the mother, and then settles the baby at the end of the feed. Although this has some advantages and involves the father in the parenting process, it can also lead to both parents becoming sleep-deprived and extremely tired! It is difficult to see the benefits of this in the long term. Coping with a new baby can be difficult enough—if both parents are tired and irritable, problems can develop.

At the risk of sounding sexist, it is worth considering whether it is sensible for both partners to have their sleep interrupted, if this means they are both tired and struggling to cope the next day. It might be more useful if at least one partner gets good sleep. If the baby is being breastfed, this will usually be the father, who will then hopefully be able to remain calm and constructive through difficult times. Although this might sound as though it is placing more workload on to the mother, there are benefits for her if the father is more rested, and therefore better able to cope with other issues. And if the father is the sole breadwinner, this makes all the more sense since he will not have the option of sleeping in or napping during the day.

Alternatively, if the baby is being bottlefed and both parents are working, then the night duties can and should be more evenly shared.

With these factors in mind, the following suggestions should help you to cope with this sometimes difficult, physically and emotionally stretching time.

Consider the pros and cons of both partners getting up throughout the night. Is it really best if you are both going to be tired and exhausted the next day? If not, decide how best to achieve a situation where at least one of you gets good sleep on a regular basis. This doesn't mean the father never helps during the night. It might be more practical for him to get up and do more of the night-time caring over the weekend when work commitments will not require him to be functioning the next day. (This suggestion is based on the assumption that in most cases, the father is working and the mother is at home more than he is, which even in the twenty-first century, remains the most common situation.)

It then becomes important to work out how the father can provide as much support and assistance in other ways. For example, if he is not going to get up in the night to help with feeding and diaper changing, can he do more of the cooking and cleaning and shopping, for example, to ease the pressures on the mother at other times? Perhaps there are things he can do to minimize disruptions during the day or evening when the mother is trying to rest or to sleep.

An exception to the golden rule of not napping during the day is early parenthood (particularly motherhood), when it is fine (and probably necessary) to rest during the day. For most mothers, it is best to sleep whenever possible! This will usually need to coincide with the baby's sleeping times. At around six months, the sleeping pattern should normalize and when the baby starts to sleep through the night, then the mother can resume her normal sleep and should avoid napping.

New parents should try to avoid over-committing themselves in the early days, weeks and months. One of the most common problems is attempting to do too much too early. This can deprive new mothers of much-needed sleep and of opportunities to nap and rest. This might even be one of the contributing factors to post-natal depression. If mothers are tired and harbor unrealistic expectations about how much they will be able to do once caught up with looking after a demanding, dependent baby, then they may well become susceptible to depression and the "baby blues."

So, work out a sensible routine with your partner and develop a system of sharing responsibilities with which you are both happy. Reduce your expectations and try not to burden yourself unnecessarily, especially in the first few months. Do less wherever possible. Your main task in these early days is to look after your child, yourself and your relationship with your partner.

Use as many of the strategies from *The Good Sleep Guide* as you can, and reassure yourself that you will get good sleep again. Babies do eventually develop their own routines and when they do, you will be able to sleep well once more. It might be hard to imagine at times, but look around and remind yourself of how many others have coped and come through relatively unscathed. If they can do it, you can too!

## Conclusion

So now you've read the book and done much more than that, I trust. You have probably made some significant and meaningful changes to your sleep routine and to your lifestyle, and are now on the way to reaping the rewards of good sleep. I hope that as your sleep has improved, so has your life. No doubt you are now feeling more energized and generally happier. Probably you are doing more and enjoying more in your life. I hope you are no longer as tired as you often were, and that if you still feel tired on occasion, you can now cope with it better, secure in the knowledge that it is a passing aberration and that you will achieve good sleep again in a night or two.

For many people, *The Good Sleep Guide* will be the start of a new life—a life of good sleeps, of more energy, enjoyment and fulfillment.

## OTHER ISSUES

This Good Sleep Program may have made you think about other areas of your life where you feel the need for improvement. Some people find that once they have realized the benefits of good sleep, they want to realize other benefits. They discover that there are significant gains to be found by resolving certain issues and by improving their psychological well being.

Most people meet at least once a year with their accountant or tax advisor and, similarly, many people have regular check-ups with their doctor and dentist. But very few people have regular consultations with a psychologist. We consult with financial advisors and lawyers when we need specialized monetary and legal advice, but we tend to talk to the hairdresser or taxi-driver about our personal problems!

I have nothing against hairdressers or taxi-drivers, but if you are having emotional problems there are many highly-qualified and experienced people (such as clinical psychologists) with expertise and professional training in applying proven treatments who can help you to substantially improve your personal life.

You don't have to just accept that things have to stay the way they are. For most people in the developed world there is no need to accept being poor or overweight. We cannot all be billionaires, but we can all learn how to save and invest wisely in order to be better off. We cannot all be fashion models (and we don't all want to be), but we can all learn to exercise and eat well to be healthy and fit. Similarly, on the emotional and psychological fronts we don't have to accept fears or anxieties that undermine our happiness and personal fulfillment. We don't have to accept insecurities and emotional obstacles that may have hampered us for some time. These problems can almost always be conquered.

By applying proven treatments and by teaching people effective skills and strategies, trained specialists, such as clinical psychologists, help people to overcome not just sleep problems, but also depression, anxiety, marital problems, and work-related stress. Perhaps your career is being held back by the fear of speaking in public, or maybe you would like to have more confidence to engage in recreational activities which you've shied away from (because of, for example, a fear of heights). By tackling these problems, people become happier and go on to be more productive in their lives and in their jobs.

In my practice, I have seen many people emerge with increased self-esteem and feel more comfortable about themselves. Not surprisingly, this often goes a long way towards an improvement in existing relationships and towards having the confidence to develop new and more rewarding relationships than they had in the past.

The people I help are not mad or crazy. They are normal people with problems experienced by many of us. They are bankers, lawyers, accountants, housewives, teachers, retirees and manual laborers. They are single and they are married. They are male and they are female. They are the average person in the street as well as the special person in the street. Some are very rich and successful. Some are struggling to get by. We can all benefit from improved emotional health. So having taken the steps to overcome the problem of broken sleep, you may now feel ready to do more for yourself to enjoy life more.

So sleep well and live well!

# INDEX